PHYSICIAN ASSISTANT

A&L's QUICK REVIEW

PHYSICIAN ASSISTANT

fourth edition

Richard R. Rahr, EdD, PA-C

Department of Physician Assistant Studies
School of Allied Health Sciences
The University of Texas Medical Branch at Galveston
Galveston, Texas

Salah Ayachi, PhD, PA-C

Department of Physician Assistant Studies
School of Allied Health Sciences
The University of Texas Medical Branch at Galveston
Galveston, Texas

Bruce R. Niebuhr, PhD

Department of Physician Assistant Studies
School of Allied Health Sciences
The University of Texas Medical Branch at Galveston
Galveston, Texas

Appleton & Lange Reviews/McGraw-Hill
Medical Publishing Division

New York Chicago San Francisco Lisbon London Madrid
Mexico City Milan New Delhi San Juan Seoul
Singapore Sydney Toronto

McGraw-Hill

*A Division of The **McGraw·Hill** Companies*

A & L's Quick Review: Physician Assistant, Fourth Edition

Copyright © 2001 by The **McGraw-Hill Companies,** Inc. All rights reserved. Printed in the United States of America. Except as permitted under the United States Copyright Act of 1976, no part of this publication may be reproduced or distributed in any form or by any means, or stored in a data base or retrieval system, without the prior written permission of the publisher.

1 2 3 4 5 6 7 8 9 0   DOC/DOC   0 9 8 7 6 5 4 3 2 1

ISBN 0-8385-0394-2

This book was set in Times by North Market Street Graphics.
The editor was Patricia Casey.
The production supervisor was Lisa Mendez.
Project management was provided by North Market Street Graphics.
The cover designer was Mary McKeon.
R.R. Donnelley & Sons was printer and binder.

This book is printed on acid-free paper.

Library of Congress Cataloging-in-Publication Data
A&L's quick review, physician assistant / [edited by] Richard R. Rahr, Salah Ayachi, Bruce R. Niebuhr.—4th ed.
    p. ; cm.
Rev. ed. of: Appleton & Lange's review for the physician assistant. 3rd ed. c1998.
Includes bibliographical references and index.
ISBN 0-8385-0394-2
    1. Physicians' assistants—Examinations, questions, etc.   I. Title: A and L's quick review, physician assistant.   II. Title: Physician assistant.   III. Rahr, Richard R.   IV. Ayachi, Salah.   V. Niebuhr, Bruce R.   VI. Appleton & Lange's review for the physician assistant.
    [DNLM: 1. Physician Assistants—Examination Questions. W 18.2 A1112 2001]
R697.P45 A67 2001
610.69'53'076 —dc21

00-068100

Contents

Contributors

Frank Ambriz, PA-C
Department of Physician Assistant Studies
The University of Texas—Pan American
Edinburg, Texas

Salah Ayachi, PhD, PA-C
Department of Physician Assistant Studies
School of Allied Health Sciences
The University of Texas Medical Branch at Galveston
Galveston, Texas

Jeff Baker, PhD
Department of Graduate Studies
School of Allied Health Sciences
The University of Texas Medical Branch at Galveston
Galveston, Texas

J. Dennis Blessing, PhD, PA-C
Department of Physician Assistant Studies
The University of Texas Health Science Center at San Antonio
San Antonio, Texas

Roberto Canales, MS, PA-C
Department of Physician Assistant Studies
School of Allied Health Sciences
The University of Texas Medical Branch at Galveston
Galveston, Texas

Marilyn R. Childers, MEd, RRT
Department of Respiratory Care
The University of Texas Medical Branch at Galveston
Galveston, Texas

Frances Coulson, MS, PA-C
Department of Physician Assistant Studies
School of Allied Health Sciences
The University of Texas Medical Branch at Galveston
Galveston, Texas

Larry Dennis, PA-C, MPAS
Physician Assistant Program
Texas Tech University
Midland, Texas

Vickie S. Etzel, PA-C
Perinatal Program
Department of Obstetrics and Gynecology
The University of Texas Medical Branch at Galveston
Galveston, Texas

Charles Haney, PA-C
Department of Neurology
Hermann Hospital
Houston, Texas

Barbara A. Lyons, MEd, PA-C
Department of Physician Assistant Studies
School of Allied Health Sciences
The University of Texas Medical Branch at Galveston
Galveston, Texas

Amy B. McAlister, PA-C
Department of Neurology
Hermann Hospital
Houston, Texas

Richard D. Muma, MPH, PA-C
Department of Physician Assistant Studies
St. Louis University
St. Louis, Missouri

Bruce R. Niebuhr, PhD
Department of Physician Assistant Studies
School of Allied Health Sciences
The University of Texas Medical Branch at Galveston
Galveston, Texas

Timothy F. Quigley, MS, PA-C
Physician Assistant Program
Wichita State University
Wichita, Kansas

Richard R. Rahr, EdD, PA-C
Department of Physician Assistant Studies
School of Allied Health Sciences
The University of Texas Medical Branch at Galveston
Galveston, Texas

Albert F. Simon, MEd, PA-C
Physician Assistant Program
Saint Francis College
Loretto, Pennsylvania

Karen S. Stephenson, MS, PA-C
Department of Physician Assistant Studies
School of Allied Health Sciences
The University of Texas Medical Branch at Galveston
Galveston, Texas

Preface

This is the fourth edition of *A & L's Quick Review: Physician Assistant*. This book is designed to aid individuals in preparing for the certification and/or recertification exams administered by the National Commission on Certification of Physician Assistants. The questions are all of the objective type and in formats similar to those found on the exams. A wide range of medical and surgical topics are covered in this edition.

Several chapters have been totally or mostly rewritten by leading physician assistant educators and practicing clinicians in various clinical specialties. The remaining chapters have been revised to include the most-up-to-date information. We wish to thank all the contributors for their hard work, and to express our gratitude to all the readers of the third edition for their suggestions and comments.

Richard R. Rahr
Salah Ayachi
Galveston, Texas

Acknowledgments

We would like to thank the staff at McGraw-Hill for their enthusiasm and support. Special thanks are due to Trish Casey for a marvelous job of smoothing out the kinks in the questions and to Stephanie Landis for making the task of reviewing the manuscript enjoyable.

1

Test-Taking Skills

Bruce R. Niebuhr, PhD
and Dennis Blessing, PhD, PA-C

Introduction

Certification and recertification are parts of the physician assistant's (PA's) professional existence. Certification is required in virtually every state and federal jurisdiction. In some places, a PA may not be able to work without certification. For this reason alone, it is important that the examination be taken seriously, using every available strategy to assure maximum achievement.

The NCCPA Examinations[1]

The Physician Assistant National Certification Examination (PANCE), the Physician Assistant National Recertification Examination (PANRE), Pathway II, and the Surgery Examination are administered by the National Commission on Certification of Physician Assistants (NCCPA).

- The PANCE is a computer-based exam consisting of 360 multiple choice questions covering basic medical and surgical knowledge.
- The PANRE is a computer-based exam consisting of 300 multiple choice questions covering basic medical and surgical knowledge.

- The Surgery Examination is a computer-based exam consisting of 180 multiple choice questions covering knowledge and skills related to surgery.
- Pathway II is a take-home exam consisting of 300 multiple choice questions covering basic medical and surgical knowledge.

All first-time takers of the examination must take the PANCE. PANCE registrants or PAs holding valid NCCPA certificates may take the optional Surgery Examination. The PANRE and Pathway II are for recertification only. All examinations are developed by independent test-writing committees composed of physician assistants and physicians from a variety of practice settings and specialties. Multiple resources and references are used, including materials from the National Board of Medical Examiners (NBME) and the Federation of State Medical Boards of the United States (FSMB). Test items are referenced and reviewed before use and are submitted to computerized analysis after use. These steps provide a degree of reliability and validity.

The NCCPA states that the examinations emphasize clinical practice. They are designed to sample a range of knowledge and skills needed for physician assistant practice. Tests, test items, and concentrations of content area may change annually. The idea is to test general physician assistant functions and specialty functions in primary care and surgery. Physical examination skills are tested in the PANCE. Certification is maintained by completing 100 hours of continuing medical education every 2 years and reexamination every 6 years. The examinations are criteria-referenced and scores are standardized.

Tests

PAs should be experienced test-takers by the time certification is needed. However, even the most experienced test-taker may approach certification and recertification with trepidation. The importance of certification as a "ticket" to practice or as an implied standard of ability, the magnitude of the information to be covered, or the costs add to the pressure to pass and be certified. The certified PA may be facing a written test for the first time since taking the certification examination or the last recertification exam. The specialty PA may fear the general content focus or lack of content in his or her area. Any number of perceptions can create anxiety and fear of the examination. Adding to these fears is the recent change in delivery to computer-based testing rather than pencil, answer sheet, and test booklet. Individual response to testing is a personal phenomenon that probably cannot be eliminated completely. However, perhaps some of the suggestions that follow will aid in minimizing anxiety and maximizing effort and will allow attainment of the best score possible.

Preparation

There is no substitute for knowledge. Preparation for the NCCPA examinations is really an ongoing event that occurs as PAs practice. However, the examination makes preparation an event and a process. Preparation for the computer-based examinations can follow a number of steps.

1. Develop a plan of study. Base the plan upon the NCCPA's "Tasks and Evaluation Objectives."[1] Write down the plan.
2. Set aside time for study well in advance of the exam.
3. Stick to your plan. Do not find excuses for not studying.
4. Although materials designed for medical students or physicians are helpful, be sure to use materials specifically developed for PAs. Summary or synopsis-type articles may be best. If you have areas of weakness, concentrate some study time in those areas.
5. Review general concepts of practice, e.g., history and physical examination, by the textbook.
6. Review a variety of materials with an emphasis on general concepts and common problems.
7. Review common EKG, chest x-ray, and laboratory findings.
8. Form study groups with other PAs.
9. Try to attend a certification or recertification continuing medical education program.
10. Practice taking tests.
11. Practice using a computer. It is not drastically different from paper tests, just a different instrument. There are computer-based review programs.
12. Do not attempt to study when you are overly tired.
13. Arrange for study time to be free of distractions and interruptions.
14. Learn some relaxation techniques. Practice and use them.

15. Send the application to the NCCPA and make a reservation at a Sylvan Technology Center.
16. Read all materials sent from the NCCPA.
17. Remember! You cannot prepare the day before the exam.

Just Before the Test

1. Review all instructions provided by the NCCPA and the Sylvan Technology Center.
2. Do not forget your scheduling permit sent to you by the NCCPA.
3. Most personal items are not allowed in the testing room. A locker is provided for prohibited personal items at the Sylvan Technology Center.
4. Have a picture ID with you. Your driver's license is best (if it has your picture).
5. Locate the Sylvan Technology Center the day before the exam. If you are testing at a site that is not familiar to you, travel a day (or two, if necessary) before the exam date and locate the site. Also, locate parking. Many test sites are in large cities where parking is always a problem.
6. Rest and get a good night's sleep the night before the exam.
7. Do not study or only do light study. Do not cram.
8. Eat breakfast. Do not overeat.
9. Dress comfortably.
10. Arrive at the site early, particularly if parking is a problem.
11. Be patient with registration personnel and the individuals giving the exam. There are procedures they are required to follow.
12. Try to relax.
13. Ask questions if you do not understand test instructions.

During the Test

1. Listen to test personnel carefully.
2. Follow directions exactly.
3. Take the opportunity to complete the brief tutorial on the computer testing system.
4. Read test directions carefully.
5. Start when told to do so.
6. The PANCE is in four blocks of 90 questions. You have 90 minutes per block.

7. Breaks are allowed between blocks.
8. Work steadily and allow 45 to 60 seconds per question.
9. All questions are in multiple choice format.
10. Answer each question as you progress. Guess, if necessary.
11. Do not fret over or spend long periods of time on questions to which you do not know the answer. Some items may be eliminated if item analysis proves they are poor questions. Some questions are trial questions and are undergoing analysis.
12. Test proctors are not allowed to answer, interpret, or clarify test questions. You must interpret questions as best you can and choose the best answer. The individuals at the testing centers are not health care professionals.
13. Try to relax. No one will know the answer to every question.

Multiple Choice Questions

Multiple choice questions are the most commonly used test question format.[2] They are the dominant type of questions on the written—and now computer-based—examinations of the NCCPA. Test-takers generally feel more comfortable with multiple choice questions because they are most familiar with this format. However, multiple choice questions can be formidable. Test-takers still need to know their material regardless of the test question type.

1. Multiple choice questions consist of two parts.
   a. The stem (a question or an incomplete statement)
   b. The alternatives—the answer (the correct choice) and the distracters (the incorrect choices)
2. The format used has four (A, B, C, D) or five (A, B, C, D, E) alternatives.
3. Our suggestions for answering multiple choice questions are as follows:
   a. Read the stem carefully.
   b. Formulate the answer in your mind.
   c. Read the answers.
   d. Select the answer that matches the answer in your mind.
4. If you do not know the answer to a question, try to eliminate some of the choices. Then choose the best answer to the best of your knowledge.
5. Use clues that may appear in the stem or alternatives. For example, "always, never, and only" should raise flags as absolutes.

6. Ultimately, if you do not know an answer, guess. If you have eliminated some of the choices, your odds when guessing have improved. The computer randomly orders the alternatives—B or C are not more likely than A, D, or E. When guessing, choose one option consistently to reduce the time you spend when guessing.
7. There is no penalty for guessing.

Following the Test

Try not to worry about your performance. The test is over. It is recommended that you not discuss the test with other takers, because it has been our experience that this creates more anxiety. Most people have difficulty recalling their answers on such a long test and any discussion may raise more doubts about performance. This creates undue worry that cannot be resolved until test results are known.

Most PAs pass the certification examination. The failure rate on the recertification examination is extremely low. The key to success for first-time takers of the certification examination is preparation beyond your PA educational process. Preparation cannot be a short-time event. We suggest that a study plan be developed and followed beginning in the year you certify or recertify.

Alternatives to the written recertification examination are being explored and may be available to some PAs. We all hope that someday the perfect evaluation tool will be created.

Conclusion

As long as certification and recertification are required and in the current format, testing is a fact of professional life. It is important to deal with it in a rational way through preparation, review, study, and practice. Your best opportunity to be successful is to approach testing as a challenge that can be met and solved.

References

1. National Commission on Certification of Physician Assistants: Available online at http://www.nccpa.net/.

2. Goltzer SZ: Taking the national board and recertification examinations: Strategies for success. *J Am Acad Phys Assist* 7(2):134–138, 1994.

2

Psychiatry

Jeff Baker, PhD

DIRECTIONS (Questions 2.1–2.45): Each of the numbered items or incomplete statements in this chapter is followed by answers or completions of the statement. Select the **one** lettered answer or completion that is **best** in each case.

2.1 The defense mechanism by which thoughts, memories, or feelings are unconsciously excluded from awareness is
  A. Regression
  B. Isolation
  C. Repression
  D. Projection
  E. Reaction formation

2.2 Adjustment disorders
  A. Cannot be treated very effectively with counseling and psychotherapy
  B. Rarely involve high levels of anxiety, depression, and/or discomfort
  C. Almost always show a clear connection to a particular, identifiable stressor
  D. Indicate a chronic and lasting pattern of poorly adapted behavior

2.3 A psychological disorder characterized by episodes of anxiety, sleeplessness, and nightmares resulting from some disturbing event in the past is called
   A. Generalized Anxiety Disorder
   B. Posttraumatic Stress Disorder
   C. Panic Disorder
   D. Manic Disorder
   E. Eating Disorder

2.4 Psychometric and neuropsychological tests are designed to
   A. Assess the human capacity to think, learn, and prosper
   B. Measure specific aspects of intelligence, thinking, and personality
   C. Assimilate factual knowledge to recall recent or remote events
   D. Determine an individual's IQ and personality style
   E. Deliver an objective measurement of innate personality and intelligence factors

2.5 Difficult patients who have obsessive personality characteristics would most likely
   A. Act as though they are superior to everyone around them
   B. Be orderly, punctual, and overly concerned with detail
   C. Fear that people want to hurt them and intend to do them harm
   D. Be isolated and solitary, detached and reclusive
   E. Have difficulty delaying gratification and may demand their discomfort be eliminated immediately

2.6 Generally, patients who are malingering
   A. Feign illness, and are often described as antisocial
   B. Are demanding, workaholic, martyrlike, and passive-aggressive
   C. Are obsessive, controlling, and perfectionistic
   D. Fear that they will never get what they want as soon as they want

2.7 Gender identity is
   A. An individual's sense of being a male or female
   B. An individual's sense of what expectation he or she has for the opposite sex
   C. Sexual behavior that is destructive to a person or people
   D. Impossible to separate out, as your impulses and parents will define what your identity will be
   E. Neither male nor female, since the hormones do not have a script for gender identity

2.8 The criteria for Sexual Aversion Disorder include all of the following **EXCEPT**
   A. Sexual acting out and permissiveness in early childhood
   B. Persistent or recurrent extreme aversion to, and avoidance of, all (or almost all) genital sexual contact with a sexual partner
   C. Marked distress or interpersonal difficulty
   D. Dysfunction that is not better accounted for by another Axis I disorder
   E. Difficulty establishing and maintaining intimate relationships

2.9 The diagnostic criteria for dyspareunia include all of the following **EXCEPT**
   A. The desire to participate in frequent sexual intercourse
   B. Recurrent or persistent genital pain associated with sexual intercourse
   C. Marked distress or interpersonal difficulty
   D. Not caused exclusively by vaginismus or lack of lubrication

2.10 All the following are major symptoms of a sleep disorder **EXCEPT**
   A. Insomnia
   B. Enuresis
   C. Hypersomnia
   D. Parasomnia
   E. Sleep-wake schedule disturbance

2.11 The Rorschach psychological assessment test, devised by Hermann Rorschach, is generally used as
   A. A structured interview of personality
   B. The projective approach to personality assessment
   C. A means of identifying a significant figure (hero) with whom subjects seem to identify
   D. A means of tapping patients' conscious associations to areas of functioning in which clinicians may be interested
   E. Stimulus words given to patients, who then respond with the first word that comes to mind

2.12 The following statement regarding sexuality and disability is **FALSE.** Individuals with spinal cord injury
   A. Have many times had their sexual function ignored by health care providers
   B. Have an interest in sexual function
   C. Are more likely to stay married than others
   D. Rarely think about or engage in sexual activity
   E. Have an incredible capacity to redirect their sexual sensitivity to other parts of their body

2.13 Which is not an adaptive function of anxiety?
   A. It prompts a person to take the necessary steps to prevent a threat or lessen its consequences.
   B. It warns of threats of bodily damage, pain, and helplessness.
   C. It helps an individual deal with social or bodily needs.
   D. It helps suppress the need to engage in trivial tasks.
   E. It prevents damage by alerting the person to carry out certain acts that forestall danger.

2.14 Depression is a product of
   A. Environmental factors
   B. Genetic factors
   C. Psychosocial factors
   D. All of the above
   E. A and B only

2.15 Schizophrenia, a psychological disorder marked by delusions, hallucinations, catatonic behavior, and flat or grossly inappropriate affect, is possibly causally related with
   A. Acetylcholine
   B. Dopamine
   C. Epinephrine
   D. Norepinephrine
   E. Both C and D

2.16 The brain region associated with auditory input, memory, encoding of new information, language comprehension, and emotions is the
   A. Temporal lobe
   B. Occipital lobe
   C. Frontal lobe
   D. Parietal lobe
   E. Cerebellum

2.17 Which is **NOT** a diagnostic criterion for Schizoid Personality Disorder?
   A. Neither desiring nor enjoying close relationships, including with family
   B. Almost always choosing solitary activities
   C. Having little, if any, interest in having sexual experiences with another person
   D. Taking pleasure in few, if any, activities
   E. Showing emotional depth and being interpersonally confident with others

2.18 In Pavlov's classical conditioning experiments, the sound of a bell could evoke salivation in dogs, even without the presentation of food. The bell sound is recognized as the
   A. Conditioned stimulus
   B. Neutral stimulus
   C. Unconditioned stimulus
   D. Unconditioned response
   E. Conditioned response

2.19 The essential feature of people with Paranoid Personality Disorder is a pervasive and unwarranted tendency to
   A. Appear to behave in an odd, eccentric, or peculiar manner
   B. Neither desire nor enjoy close relationships, including being part of a family

C. Have odd beliefs or magical thinking inconsistent with subcultural norms
D. Show disregard for the law and violation of the rights of others beginning at age 15
E. Interpret other people's actions as deliberately demeaning or threatening

2.20 John is an individual who has a pervasive pattern of instability in his interpersonal relationships. He has chronic feelings of emptiness, displays inappropriately intense anger, is involved in physical fights, and impulsively participates in spending, sex, and reckless driving. Based on this information, which best describes John's personality disorder?
A. Paranoid
B. Cyclothymic
C. Borderline
D. Schizotypal
E. Dependent

2.21 Which is an incorrect statement regarding the influence of psychological factors on a patient's medical condition?
A. Many times, they delay recovery.
B. They interfere with medical treatment.
C. They constitute additional health risks for the individual.
D. They tend to positively assist the patient in coping with chronic conditions.

2.22 Which of the following is **NOT** an important aspect of working with chronic pain patients? As a health care professional, you are to
A. Explain the nature of the pain signal
B. Explain realistic expectations about the degree and course of pain
C. Explain that pain is all in the head
D. Maximize the placebo effect by making the initial doses large rather than small, supporting belief in efficacy, and suggestion through your attitude about administering the analgesic
E. Relieve concomitant anxiety, if necessary

2.23 Which of the following is **NOT** true about tardive dyskinesia?
  A. It is a delayed effect of antipsychotic medications.
  B. It rarely occurs until after 6 mo of treatment.
  C. It consists of abnormal, involuntary, irregular choreo-athetoid movements.
  D. It is managed through prevention, diagnosis, and treatment.
  E. It is least likely to occur in patients taking dopamine receptor antagonists chronically.

2.24 A maltreated child often shows no obvious signs of being battered, but has multiple minor physical evidence of emotional—and, at times, nutritional—deprivation, neglect, and abuse. A typical history of maltreated children will **NOT** include
  A. History of failure to thrive
  B. Weight and height above the 75th percentile of normal
  C. Malnutrition
  D. Poor skin hygiene
  E. Irritability and withdrawal

2.25 Many individuals have difficulty coping with sexual assault. A rape survivor may do best in recovering from the trauma if he or she
  A. Never directly talks about it
  B. Waits 6 mo before addressing it
  C. Receives immediate support for it
  D. Pursues legal action
  E. Waits 12 mo before talking about it

2.26 Which of the following is **NOT** an indicator of child sexual abuse?
  A. Contradictions made by the child about the story and circumstances
  B. The presence of STDs in the child
  C. Retractions of previous accusations made by the child
  D. The child's knowledge of sexuality and acting out sexually
  E. The ability of the child to correctly name his or her body parts

2.27 Which of the following is a **TRUE** statement?
   A. Oppositional Defiant Disorder (ODD) is nearly identical to ADHD, except ODD children do not exhibit attention or concentration problems.
   B. About 40% of children with Tourette's disorder have ADHD and/or Obsessive-Compulsive Disorder as well.
   C. The majority of disruptive disorders have a known organic etiology.
   D. Children exposed to sexual abuse never perpetrate abuse on others.

2.28 Which of the following is **NOT** necessary for a child to be diagnosed with Major Depressive Disorder?
   A. Feelings of worthlessness
   B. Diminished ability to think or concentrate
   C. Social or academic impairment
   D. Daily insomnia or hypersomnia
   E. Previous suicide attempt

2.29 Which of the following is **MOST** predictive of suicidal ideation in children?
   A. Depressed or irritable mood
   B. Verbalizations of hopelessness
   C. Presence of peer conflict
   D. Presence of family conflict
   E. Presence of spiritual conflict

2.30 According to Freud, the mental structure that mediates conflicts between unconscious impulses and external reality is the
   A. Ego
   B. Id
   C. Preconscious
   D. Superego

2.31 Neurons are polarized, elongated cells that are uniquely capable of instantaneous, intercellular communication. Which of the following is **NOT** true?
  A. Each neuron is polarized with respect to transmission of information.
  B. Neurons are made up of the gray matter within the brain and are responsible for all executive functions except speech and movement.
  C. Neurons receive information in the form of extracellular signals.
  D. There are two broad classes of neurons: interneurons and projection neurons.
  E. The collections of neuronal cell bodies within the nervous system constitute the gray matter.

2.32 Which is not part of a comprehensive workup of dementia?
  A. Physical exam with vital signs
  B. Mental status exam
  C. Review of medications and blood and urine screens with a physiological workup
  D. Spine evaluation, including the Hoover test
  E. Neuropsychological testing

2.33 About what percentage of schizophrenics recover?
  A. <1
  B. 100
  C. 10
  D. 33
  E. 80

2.34 Which term refers to a generalized fear of practically everything without knowing what causes this fear?
  A. Phobia
  B. Panic attack
  C. Stressing out
  D. Melancholia
  E. Anxiety

2.35 Axis II of the DSM-IV consists of
  A. Clinical disorders
  B. Global assessment of functioning
  C. Psychosocial and environmental problems
  D. General medical conditions
  E. Personality disorders and mental retardation

2.36 A true statement about anorexia nervosa is
  A. The individual refuses to maintain weight loss.
  B. The individual refuses to maintain a minimum normal weight, has an intense fear of gaining weight, and significantly misinterprets the body and its shape.
  C. There are no biologic, social, or psychological factors implicated in the cause.
  D. It is based on endogenous endorphins contributing to hunger.
  E. The onset usually occurs between ages 3 and 10.

2.37 The Minnesota Multiphasic Personality Inventory (MMPI) has 10 clinical scales and three validity scales. It is an example of what kind of test?
  A. An objective measure of personality
  B. A projective measure of personality
  C. A psychopathic deviate analysis of behavior
  D. A measure of chronic pain and inkblot measures
  E. A representation of 10 thematic pictures

2.38 Anorexia nervosa
  A. Is 10 to 20 times more prevalent in females than in males
  B. Occurs in 4% of adolescent girls
  C. Is more common in upper than in lower economic classes
  D. Occurs most often in young women in food preparation professions

2.39 Which of the following diagnostic criteria for schizophrenia is **NOT** important according to the DSM-IV?

A. At least two of the following: delusions, hallucinations, disorganized speech, grossly disorganized or catatonic behavior, and/or negative symptoms (affective flattening, alogia, or avolition) are present.

B. The individual exhibits social/occupational dysfunction.

C. Continuous signs of the disturbance persist for at least 6 mo.

D. The symptoms have a significant degree of impact on the individual's ego functioning.

E. It is not related to a general medical condition or substance use/abuse.

2.40 Even though clonidine has major indications in psychiatry, it is **NOT** primarily used for

A. Memory retrieval

B. Control of withdrawal symptoms of opiates

C. Treatment of Tourette's disorder

D. Control of aggressive behavior in children

E. Control of hyperactive behavior in children

2.41 In the U.S., spouse abuse is estimated to occur in 2 million to 12 million families. This form of domestic violence has received attention because of the civil rights and feminist movements, even though the problem is of long standing. The major concern in spouse abuse is

A. Physical abuse by the husband

B. Physical abuse by the wife

C. Sexual abuse of children

D. Physical abuse of parents

2.42 A comprehensive evaluation of a child includes all of the following **EXCEPT**

A. Interviews with the child, parents, and family

B. Obtaining information regarding the child's current school functioning

C. Assessment of the physician-patient relationship

D. Assessment of the child's intellectual functioning

E. Assessment of the child's academic achievement

2.43 All of the following are different syndromes in mental retardation **EXCEPT**
  A. Down syndrome
  B. Fragile X syndrome
  C. Prader-Willi syndrome
  D. Apgar syndrome
  E. Cat's cry syndrome

2.44 In the movie *As Good as It Gets,* Jack Nicholson plays a character who spends an inordinate amount of time checking and rechecking that his door is locked and then goes through a ritual of locking it a certain number of times each time. The best characterization of this personality trait is
  A. Intermittent Explosive Disorder
  B. Major Depressive Disorder
  C. Obsessive-Compulsive Disorder
  D. Factitious Disorder
  E. Multiple Personality Disorder

2.45 Which one of the following is **TRUE** of the differences between male and female sexuality?
  A. Males have a built-in capacity to be multiorgasmic.
  B. Females have no refractory period.
  C. Males have 98% the same genetic makeup as chimpanzees and both believe that foreplay is a total waste of time.
  D. 98% of females believe that penis size is what matters.
  E. Explicit sexual fantasies are common only to normal men and abnormal women.

Psychiatry

Answers and Discussion

2.1 **(C)** The defense mechanism involved with assisting an individual to put away thoughts and uncomfortable memories is known as repression. It involves expelling or withholding from consciousness an idea or feeling. Primary repression refers to the curbing of ideas and feelings before they have attained consciousness; secondary repression excludes from awareness what was once experienced at a conscious level. The repressed is not really forgotten in that symbolic behavior may be present. Conscious perception of instincts and feelings is blocked in repression. (*1, pp 218–220*)

2.2 **(C)** Adjustment disorders usually have a direct component of a specific stressor, for example a change in a medical condition such as diabetes, stroke, or cardiac problems. The individual can usually identify the stressor that is responsible for the adjustment problem. Adjustment disorders are one of the most common psychiatric diagnoses for disorders of patients hospitalized for medical and surgical problems. In one study, 5% of people admitted to a hospital over a 3-year period were classified as having an adjustment disorder. In a survey of psychiatric patients, 10% of the sample population were found to have an adjustment disorder. (*1, pp 770–774*)

2.3 (B) Posttraumatic Stress Disorder is closely associated with an individual experiencing anxiety, difficulty with sleep, and sometimes nightmares as a result of a traumatic event. The stress causing Posttraumatic Stress Disorder is overwhelming enough to affect almost anyone. It can arise from experiences in war, torture, natural catastrophes, assault, rape, or serious accidents—for example, in cars and burning buildings. People reexperience the traumatic event in their dreams and their daily thoughts; they are determined to evade anything that would bring the event to mind. Other symptoms are depression, anxiety, and cognitive difficulties such as poor concentration. (*1, pp 617–623*)

2.4 (B) Psychometrics assist the clinician in obtaining the individual's thinking ability (intelligence and problem-solving ability) as well as personality factors. Psychiatric tests are not always required to assess psychiatric symptoms, but they are extremely valuable in determining an individual's intellectual functioning, academic difficulties, and objective assessment of personality variables. (*1, pp 1133–1136*)

2.5 (B) Obsessive-compulsive individuals tend to be very orderly with their possessions and self-care, are very conscientious of being late, and are many times preoccupied with details to the point that it interferes with work or pleasure activities. The disorder is characterized by emotional constriction, orderliness, perseverance, stubbornness, and indecisiveness. The essential feature is a pervasive pattern of perfectionism and inflexibility. (*1, pp 609–617*)

2.6 (A) Malingering patients have no specific cause of their illness and are usually motivated by secondary gain such as financial reward or relief from responsibility (work). Many times they develop an antisocial personality characteristic. (*1, pp 860–861*)

2.7 (A) Your gender identity refers to your sense of being a male or female. Many times this is confused as the individual is going through early developmental stages. Gender role and gender are related yet different concepts. Gender role refers to stereotypical behaviors; gender is the biologic determination of maleness or femaleness. (*1, pp 711–719*)

2.8 (A) Sexual aversion has little or nothing to do with acting out or permissiveness in childhood. It is a persistent or recurrent extreme aversion to, and avoidance of, all (or almost all) genital sexual contact with a sexual partner. (*1, pp 684–685*)

2.9 (A) It is very unusual for an individual to have the desire to frequently participate in sexual intercourse if he or she is experiencing dyspareunia. Dyspareunia is recurrent or persistent genital pain occurring in either men or women before, during, or after intercourse. It is much more common in women than men and is often related to and coincident with vaginismus. (*1, p 690*)

2.10 (B) Enuresis is not a component of most sleep disorders. Insomnia, hypersomnia, parasomnia, and sleep-wake disturbances are components of sleep disorders. (*1, pp 741–759*)

2.11 (B) The Rorschach is a projective approach to personality assessment. It does not rely on a structured interview. It does not include an attempt to identify a hero with whom the subject identifies (Thematic Apperception test). It is not designed to tap the patient's conscious associations (free association), nor does it use stimulus words. (*1, p 197*)

2.12 (D) Individuals with SCI have the same sexual thoughts and desires as they held previous to the injury. (*2, p 57*)

2.13 (D) Many times individuals have an overwhelming need to participate in trivial tasks in an attempt to ignore anxiety. When considered simply as an alerting signal, anxiety seems to be basically the same emotion as fear. As a warning of an external or internal threat, anxiety has lifesaving qualities. It prompts a person to take the necessary steps to prevent a threat or to lessen its consequences. (*1, pp 581–628*)

2.14 (D) Environmental, genetic, and psychosocial factors all play roles in the development of depression. Depression is the psychological symptom that has been most associated with disruptions in biologic rhythms. Early morning awakening, decreased latency of rapid-eye-movement (REM) sleep, and neuroendocrine perturbations that are seen in depression can all be conceptualized as reflecting a disorder of coordination in biologic rhythms. (*1, pp 525–528*)

2.15 **(B)** Dopamine is the neurotransmitter that appears to have a causal association with schizophrenia. The dopaminergic axon terminal is the site of synthesis for dopamine. Dopamine is one of the three catecholamine neurotransmitters synthesized starting with the amino acid tyrosine. The other two catecholamine neurotransmitters are norepinephrine and epinephrine. (*1, pp 111–113*)

2.16 **(A)** The temporal lobe is the brain region most associated with auditory function, memory, information encoding, language comprehension, and emotions. (*1, pp 93–94*)

2.17 **(E)** Individuals with Schizoid Personality Disorder rarely have emotional depth or any confidence in interpersonal relationships. The disorder is diagnosed in patients who display a lifelong pattern of social withdrawal. Their discomfort with human interaction, their introversion, and their bland, constricted affect are noteworthy. Individuals with Schizoid Personality Disorder are often seen by others as eccentric, isolated, or lonely. (*1, pp 782–783*)

2.18 **(A)** In classical conditioning, the sound of the bell in this example is the conditioned stimulus that evokes the salivation in the dog. (*1, pp 148–149*)

2.19 **(E)** An individual with Paranoid Personality Disorder usually interprets other people's actions as deliberately demeaning or threatening. (*1, pp 780–782*)

2.20 **(C)** Individuals who are classified as having Borderline Personality Disorder frequently suffer chronic feelings of emptiness, display inappropriate intense anger, and are involved in physical altercations and other impulsive behaviors. (*1, pp 786–787*)

2.21 (D) Psychopathologic factors tend to have a negative effect on most patients and will delay or exacerbate a medical condition such as stress-related behaviors, arrhythmia, hypertension, or tension headache. (*1, pp 119–121*)

2.22 (C) Patients with chronic pain have probably already been told by someone that "the pain is all in your head." There is no good reason for stating this to the patient. It does not help the rapport with the patient and may decrease adherence to a treatment protocol. It is best to acknowledge the pain as that individual's experience and to develop an effective intervention plan. (*1, pp 641–644*)

2.23 (E) The longer patients take dopamine receptor antagonists, the more likely they are to experience tardive dyskinesia. Tardive dyskinesia is a delayed effect of antipsychotics; it rarely occurs until after 6 mo of treatment. The disorder consists of abnormal, involuntary, irregular choreoathetoid movements of the muscles of the head, limbs, and trunk. (*1, pp 485–486*)

2.24 (B) It is unusual for the maltreated child to be at or above the 75th percentile in height and weight. It is more typical that the child has a history of failure to thrive and malnutrition. Failure-to-thrive syndromes have been traced to negative attachment experiences. Attachment disorders are characterized by biopsychosocial pathology that results from maternal deprivation or a lack of care by and interaction with the mother or a significant caregiver. (*1, p 147*)

2.25 (C) Immediate support is an important aspect of sexual assault treatment. Most hospitals have a sexual assault survivor response team that assists in identifying support networks. (*1, pp 854–855*)

2.26 (E) Naming body parts is not typically an indicator of child sexual abuse. Most parents are encouraged to be open and honest about the correct naming of body parts, including the genitalia. (*1, pp 849–851*)

2.27 (B) Tourette's is correlated with ADHD and/or OCD in children. Tourette's disorder causes distress or significant impairment in important areas of functioning. The disorder has an onset before the age of 18 years, and it is not caused by substances or by a general medical condition. (*1, pp 1215–1220*)

2.28 (E)   A suicide attempt is not a requirement for the diagnosis of Major Depressive Disorder in children. In many cases, the onset of depression occurs in children who have had several years of difficulties with hyperactivity, Separation Anxiety Disorder, or intermittent depressive symptoms. Major Depressive Disorder in children is diagnosed most easily when it is acute and occurs in a child without previous psychological symptoms. (*1, pp 1246–1247*)

2.29 (C)   Conflict in peer relationships is the best predictor out of this list of possibilities. The suicide rate among adolescents has quadrupled since 1950, from 2.5 to 11.2 per 100,000 adolescents. Suicide currently accounts for 12% of deaths in the adolescent age group. The most common method of completed suicide in children and adolescents is the use of firearms, which accounts for about two-thirds of all suicides in boys and almost one-half of suicides in girls. The second most common method of suicide in boys is hanging; in girls, about one-fourth commit suicide through ingestion of toxic substances. (*1, pp 1250–1252*)

2.30 (A)   The ego mediates between the id (sometimes referred to as the child within) and the superego (sometimes referred to as the adult). (*1, pp 217–218*)

2.31 (B)   Neurons are not made up of gray matter, gray matter is made up of neurons. Neurons are responsible for all intracellular communication and are involved in the executive functions of speech and movement. (*1, p 76*)

2.32 (D)   The spine is an important component in a physical examination but not specifically related to dementia. Dementia is characterized by multiple cognitive defects that include impairment in memory without impairment in consciousness. The cognitive functions that can be affected include general intelligence, learning and memory, language, problem solving, orientation, perception, attention and concentration, judgment, and social abilities. Personality is also affected. The Hoover test sometimes identifies malingering in low back pain. (*1, pp 328–345*)

2.33 (D) About one-third of those individuals diagnosed with schizophrenia seem to recover. Schizophrenia is described as a disturbance that lasts for at least 6 mo and includes at least 1 mo of active-phase symptoms. There are a number of theories regarding the development and onset of schizophrenia including stress, biologic factors, and psychosocial factors. All apparently contribute. (*1, pp 504–508*)

2.34 (E) Anxiety is the best answer as it refers to a generalized state. Phobia refers to a specific object or situation, as does a panic attack. A phobia is defined as an irrational fear that produces a conscious avoidance of the feared subject, activity, or situation. Phobic reactions usually disrupt people's ability to function. (*1, pp 603–609*)

2.35 (E) Axis II refers to personality disorders and mental retardation. Axis I refers to clinical disorders, Axis III refers to medical condition, Axis IV refers to psychosocial stressors, and Axis V refers to general adaptive functioning. (*1, pp 287–305*)

2.36 (B) Anorexia nervosa is a condition in which the individual refuses to maintain normal body weight, has a distorted body image, and fears gaining weight. Biologic, social, and psychological factors are implicated as causes of anorexia nervosa. (*1, pp 720–727*)

2.37 (A) The MMPI or MMPI-2 is an objective measure of personality and consists of 567 true/false items standardized on clinical populations. It is used by psychologists to obtain additional objective data to confirm or rule out possible psychological disorders. (*1, p 195*)

2.38 (A) Anorexia nervosa is estimated to occur in only 0.5% to 1% of adolescent girls, more frequently in developing countries, and in greatest frequency among young women in professions requiring thinness. (*1, p 720*)

2.39 (D) While ego functioning is important in the development and maintenance of self, it is not a criterion on which a diagnosis of schizophrenia is made. In the United States, the lifetime prevalence of schizophrenia has been variously reported as ranging from 1 to 1.5%. Although two-thirds of treated patients require hospitalization, only about half of all patients with schizophrenia obtain treatment, in spite of the severity of the disorder. (*1, p 457*)

2.40 (A) Clonidine is effective in reducing the autonomic symptoms of opiate and opioid withdrawal. Some clinicians use clonidine as a first-line drug to treat Tourette's disorder instead of the standard drugs haloperidol (Haldol) and pimozide (Orap) because of the serious adverse effects associated with these antipsychotics. Clonidine is a third-line agent for treating pure ADHD, after the sympathomimetics and the antidepressants. Clonidine has not been identified as an agent that facilitates memory retrieval. (*1, pp 1015–1016*)

2.41 (A) The major problem in spouse abuse is wife abuse. Wife beating occurs in every racial and religious background and in all socioeconomic strata, and is most frequent in families with problems of substance abuse. Several factors are said to contribute to this problem, including behavioral, cultural, psychologic, and interpersonal factors. (*1, p 853*)

2.42 (C) Although the relationship between the physician and patient is important, it is not evaluated as part of the diagnostic criteria for any disorder. (*1, pp 3–11*)

2.43 (D) The Apgar is the scale used to evaluate newborn infants and not a syndrome in mental retardation. Mental retardation is the overriding feature of Down syndrome. Most people with the syndrome are moderately to severely retarded, with only a minority having an IQ above 50. People with Down syndrome tend to show marked deterioration in language, memory, self-care skills, and problem-solving in their thirties. Fragile X syndrome is the second most common single cause of mental retardation. The syndrome results from a mutation on the X chromosome at what is known as the fragile site. Prader-Willi syndrome is postulated to be the result of a small deletion involving chromosome 15, usually occurring sporadically. Cat's cry syndrome occurs in children who lack part of chromosome 5. They are severely retarded and show many signs often associated with chromosomal aberrations, such as microcephaly, low-set ears, oblique palpebral fissures, hypertelorism, and micrognathia. The characteristic catlike cry caused by laryngeal abnormalities, which gave the syndrome its name, gradually changes and disappears with increasing age. (*1, pp 1137–1154*)

2.44 (C)   Jack Nicholson plays a cantankerous man who has a creative side but also clearly demonstrates obsessive-compulsive traits such as repetitive checking (locking the door) and ritualistic behaviors (not stepping on cracks in the sidewalk). (*1, pp 609–617*)

2.45 (B)   Females have no refractory period and are capable of responding to sexual stimulation immediately following orgasm. Even though males (and female humans) have 98% the same genetic makeup as chimpanzees, male humans do participate in sexual stimulation (foreplay) before sexual intercourse; chimpanzees do not. Males can be multiorgasmic, but as a general rule it is not a built in feature. The majority of females do not believe that penis size is most important. Sexual fantasies are experienced by both normal males and normal females. (*1, pp 685–687*)

References

1. Kaplan KI, Sadock BJ: *Synopsis of Psychiatry: Behavioral Sciences/Clinical Psychiatry,* 8/e, Baltimore, Williams & Wilkins, 1998.

2. Ducharme SH, Gill KM: *Sexuality After Spinal Cord Injury,* Baltimore, Brookes, 1997.

3

Asthma and Allergy

Karen S. Stephenson, MS, PA-C

DIRECTIONS (Questions 3.1–3.20): Each of the numbered items or incomplete statements in this chapter is followed by answers or completions of the statement. Select the **one** lettered answer or completion that is **best** in each case.

3.1 Which of the following is **NOT** a symptom of asthma?
 A. Breathlessness
 B. Chest tightness
 C. Coughing
 D. Sneezing

3.2 Which is **NOT** characteristic of asthma in children under the age of 5 years?
 A. History of recurrent bronchospasms
 B. History of cough that worsens at night
 C. History of seborrheic dermatitis
 D. History of allergic rhinitis in the immediate family

3.3 When evaluating a patient for signs of asthma, you are likely to find each of the following **EXCEPT**
 A. Hyperresonant chest percussion
 B. Nasal secretions
 C. Prolonged expiration of breath sounds
 D. Rales

3.4 Which of the following is most likely to precipitate an asthma episode in an infant?
A. Influenza virus
B. Parainfluenza virus
C. Respiratory syncytial virus
D. Rhinovirus

3.5 When is an asthmatic exacerbation at its worst?
A. 3 to 4 A.M.
B. 1 to 2 A.M.
C. 11 P.M. to 12 A.M.
D. 9 to 10 P.M.

3.6 All of the following should be included in the differential diagnosis for asthma **EXCEPT**
A. Congenital anomalies of the respiratory tract
B. Cystic fibrosis
C. Foreign body aspiration
D. Neurofibromatosis

3.7 Which of the following oxygen saturation readings would indicate a severe exacerbation of asthma?
A. 99%
B. 95%
C. 91%
D. 90%

3.8 All of the following findings are likely to be present during an acute severe exacerbation of asthma **EXCEPT**
A. Peak expiratory flow rate 90% of normal for patient
B. Pulsus paradoxus of 20 to 40 mm Hg
C. Elevated respiratory rate
D. Cyanotic skin color

3.9 Treatment for an acute exacerbation of asthma includes all of the following **EXCEPT**
A. High-dose inhaled steroid
B. Long-acting β_2 agonist
C. Oral steroids
D. Prophylactic antibiotics

3.10 All of the following anti-inflammatory medications are recommended for the treatment of mild persistent asthma **EXCEPT**
A. Cromolyn
B. Inhaled steroid
C. Nedocromil
D. Theophylline

3.11 If your pediatric patient develops an acute asthma exacerbation, all of the following should be initiated **EXCEPT**
A. Begin β agonist with two to four puffs at 20-min intervals
B. Begin oral steroid at 10 to 20 mg/kg/day
C. Consult clinician concerning exacerbation
D. Follow peak expiratory flow rate carefully

3.12 Which of the following statements about allergic rhinitis is **NOT** true?
A. Cytokines lead to inflammation and nasal congestion.
B. Histamines lead to edema and mucous production.
C. IgM initiates the allergic response to antigens.
D. Pollens are a common cause of allergic rhinitis.

3.13 Symptoms of perennial allergic rhinitis in children may include all of the following **EXCEPT**
A. Frequent colds
B. Itchy palate and throat
C. Poor school performance
D. Snoring during sleep

3.14 Which is **NOT** a physical sign of allergic rhinitis?
A. Boggy mucosa
B. Enlarged turbinates
C. Reddened mucosa
D. Serous nasal discharge

3.15 Dennie lines are wrinkles on the
A. Bridge of the nose
B. Lower eyelids
C. Upper lip
D. Nasal mucosa

3.16 Which of the following stains is used to identify eosinophils in nasal mucus?
   A. Gram stain
   B. Hansel stain
   C. Tzanck stain
   D. Wright stain

3.17 Which of the following is **NOT** a component of vasomotor rhinitis?
   A. Normal eye exam
   B. Elevated IgE levels
   C. Prominent nasal congestion
   D. Poor response to antihistamines

3.18 Appropriate treatment of allergic rhinitis should include all of the following **EXCEPT**
   A. α-adrenergic agents
   B. Antihistamines
   C. Encasement of bedding
   D. Filtering of inside air

3.19 Which of the following medications for asthma may affect linear growth?
   A. Corticosteroids
   B. Cromolyn
   C. Leukotrienes
   D. Theophylline

3.20 Which is **NOT** true of exercise-induced asthma?
   A. It is suggested by cough, chest tightness, or wheezing during exercise.
   B. It may also induce a 15% drop in FEV post exercise.
   C. Assessment should include a 10-min warmup
   D. It is treated with a steroid MDI

Asthma and Allergy

Answers and Discussion

3.1 **(D)**   Sneezing is a symptom of allergic rhinitis or viral respiratory infections, both of which can commonly precipitate an asthmatic episode. (*1, p 2*)

3.2 **(C)**   Children and adults with asthma can have a history of atopic dermatitis rather than seborrheic dermatitis. This rash is scaly but rough and occurs beyond the distribution of seborrheic dermatitis. (*1, p 4*)

3.3 **(D)**   Rales point toward infection or congestive heart failure rather than asthma. Rhonchi and/or wheezing are more likely with asthma. (*1, p 4*)

3.4 **(C)**   Respiratory syncytial virus is the most likely infectious cause of asthma episodes in infants and is strongly associated with the development of asthma. The other viruses are more common in older children and adults. (*2, pp 1190–1191*)

3.5 **(A)**   Exacerbations of asthma tend to be worst at 3 to 4 A.M. At that time circadian rhythms bring about bronchoconstriction. Because of this, care must be taken to ask about nocturnal symptoms even if the patient with asthma is doing well during the day. (*3, p 257*)

34

3.6 (D) All but neurofibromatosis should be included in the differential diagnosis for asthma, especially in that wheezing in children may result from congenital heart disease. (*2, p 1192*)

3.7 (D) An oxygen saturation reading of less than 90% indicates severe respiratory compromise and requires immediate intervention. (*2, p 1191*)

3.8 (B) Peak expiratory flow rate is usually 50% or less of expected normal during a severe exacerbation of asthma. (*2, p 1191*)

3.9 (D) High-dose inhaled steroids, long-acting β_2 agonists, and oral steroids are recommended for severe, persistent asthma. Antibiotics should be reserved for identified infections. (*1, p 11*)

3.10 (D) All but theophylline are recommended for mild, persistent asthma, defined as asthma with daytime symptoms 3 to 6 times per week and nocturnal symptoms 3 to 4 times per month. Peak expiratory flow rate remains at or greater than 80% of predicted value for patient. (*1, pp 10–11*)

3.11 (B) Begin prednisone at 1 to 2 mg/kg/day for 3 to 10 days at a maximum of 60 mg/day. The steroid should be continued until the PEFR returns to 80% of normal or personal best (*1, p 36*)

3.12 (C) IgE triggers the allergic response to many allergens, including pollens, animal dander, molds, and dust mites. (*4, p 1179*)

3.13 (B) Other symptoms of perennial allergic rhinitis include recurrent otitis media, nasal speech, fatigue, malaise, mouth breathing, and epistaxis. Sneezing, on the other hand, is more common in acute seasonal allergic rhinitis; other symptoms include itchy palate and throat, headaches, and itchy tearing eyes. Both types cause rhinorrhea, usually clear. Children under the age of 6 years usually have the perennial type; those over 6 have more acute symptoms. (*4, p 1179*)

3.14 (C) Mucosal changes in allergic rhinitis result in pale mucosa, whereas viral infection results in reddened mucosa. (*4, p 33*)

3.15 (B) Dennie lines are extra lines on the lower eyelid in persons with allergic rhinitis. (*4, p 62*)

3.16 (B) Hansel stain can be used to identify eosinophils in the nasal mucus. (*4, p 1180*)

3.17 (B) Vasomotor rhinitis may mimic perennial allergic rhinitis, but does not involve an allergic response to nasal irritants. (*4, p 1180*)

3.18 (A) α-adrenergic agents can lead to rebound congestion if used for more than several days. (*4, p 1180*)

3.19 (A) Linear growth may also be affected by poor asthma control. (*1, p 14*)

3.20 (D) Exercise-induced asthma is most often treated with short-acting β agonist 5 to 60 min before exercise. (*1, p 15*)

References

1. National, Heart, Lung, and Blood Institute: *Practical Guide for the Diagnosis and Management of Asthma,* NIH Publication No. 96-4053, Bethesda, MD, National Institutes of Health, 1997.

2. Fireman P: Asthma. In: Hoekelman RA, Friedman SB, Nelson NM, Seidel HM, et al (eds): *Primary Pediatric Care,* 3/e, St. Louis, Mosby-Year Book, pp 1190–1195, 1997.

3. Stauffer JL. Lung. In: Tierney LM, McPhee SJ, Papadakis MA (eds): *Current Medical Diagnosis & Treatment,* 37/e, Stamford, CT, Appleton & Lange, 1998.

4. Schuberth KC: Allergic rhinitis. In: Hoekelman RA, Friedman SB, Nelson NM, Seidel HM, et al (eds): *Primary Pediatric Care,* 3/e, St. Louis, Mosby-Year Book, pp 1179–1181, 1997.

4

HIV/AIDS

Richard D. Muma, MPH, PA-C

DIRECTIONS (Questions 4.1–4.40): Each of the numbered items or incomplete statements in this chapter is followed by answers or completions of the statement. Select the **one** lettered answer or completion that is **best** in each case.

4.1 All of the following symptoms describe the presentation of Kaposi's sarcoma in the AIDS patient **EXCEPT** which?
   A. It begins as tiny macular violaceous lesion.
   B. It is commonly found on the skin.
   C. It may be associated with signs of lymphatic obstruction.
   D. Skin lesions are usually painful.

4.2 In adults and adolescents, which of the following diseases are diagnostic of AIDS?
   A. Candidiasis of the esophagus, trachea, bronchi, or lungs
   B. Kaposi's sarcoma in a patient less than 60 years of age
   C. *Pneumocystis carinii* pneumonia
   D. Pulmonary *Mycobacterium tuberculosis*
   E. All of the above

4.3 Defects commonly seen in the immune system when associated with HIV infection include all of the following **EXCEPT**
   A. Abnormal B-cell function
   B. Increased chemotaxis
   C. Decreased parasite killing
   D. Decreased response to soluble antigen

4.4 A 23-year-old Latin American man presents in your office complaining of shortness of breath, a dry hacking cough, and a temperature of 40°C. On questioning, the patient gives a history of intravenous drug use and a positive HIV test 1 year ago. Which of the following should be included in your differential diagnoses?
   A. Cytomegalovirus (CMV) pneumonitis
   B. Viral pneumonia
   C. *P. carinii* pneumonia
   D. Pulmonary tuberculosis
   E. All of the above

4.5 In an HIV-1 positive patient, a chest x-ray showing diffuse bilateral interstitial infiltrates supports which of the following diagnoses?
   A. Pulmonary embolus
   B. *Klebsiella pneumoniae* pneumonia
   C. *Streptococcus pneumoniae* pneumonia
   D. *P. carinii* pneumonia

4.6 Kaposi's sarcoma commonly presents in the
   A. Central nervous system
   B. Skin
   C. Bone
   D. Retina

4.7 Goals of the clinical evaluation of patients infected with HIV include
   A. Rapid identification of all treatable infectious diseases
   B. Consideration of experimental measures
   C. Evaluation of the immune system
   D. Initiation of approved anti-HIV therapy
   E. All of the above

4.8 Which of the following should be present before antiretroviral agents are started in asymptomatic HIV-infected adults?
  A. CD4 count ≤ 500 cells per cubic millimeter
  B. More than 20,000 (RT-PCR) copies of HIV RNA per milliliter
  C. Willingness of patient to be treated
  D. A and B only
  E. A, B, and C

4.9 When conducting a history on an individual infected with HIV, all of the following would be beneficial to know **EXCEPT**
  A. A comprehensive review of systems
  B. A history of sexually transmitted diseases
  C. HIV risk factors
  D. Allergies as a child

4.10 Causes of pulmonary pathology in the AIDS patient include all of the following **EXCEPT**
  A. Vacuolar myelopathy
  B. Cryptococcosis
  C. *P. carinii*
  D. Coccidioidomycosis

4.11 A 39-year-old white man who is HIV positive and has a CD4 count of less than 200 per cubic millimeter presents with a 2-day history of increased dizziness on ambulation, left-sided weakness, severe frontal headaches, and fevers. All of the following should be included in the differential diagnosis **EXCEPT**
  A. Brainstem lymphoma
  B. Cryptococcal meningitis
  C. Toxoplasma encephalitis
  D. AIDS dementia complex

4.12 Laboratory tests that may be helpful to determine the progression of HIV infection include
  A. β_2-microglobulin
  B. HIV-ELISA
  C. CD4 count
  D. Viral load
  E. All of the above

4.13 Which of the following is useful in the treatment of *P. carinii* pneumonia?
  A. Amphotericin B
  B. Sulfadiazine
  C. 5-flucytosine
  D. Trimethoprim/sulfamethoxazole

4.14 Treatment options for oral candidiasis include
  A. Nystatin
  B. Clotrimazole
  C. Ketoconazole
  D. Fluconazole
  E. All of the above

4.15 Adverse effects of protease inhibitors include
  A. Anemia
  B. Blue nail pigmentation
  C. Abnormal fat distribution
  D. Granulocytopenia

4.16 Treatment options for cytomegalovirus retinitis include
  A. Trimethoprim/sulfamethoxazole
  B. Trimethoprim-dapsone
  C. Pentamidine isethionate
  D. Ganciclovir

4.17 The initial laboratory workup of asymptomatic adult patients at risk for HIV includes which of the following?
  A. Serology for CMV, EBV, HSV, and toxoplasma
  B. HIV-ELISA and Western blot confirmation
  C. CD4 count
  D. HIV viral load

4.18 Acute cryptococcal meningitis may be treated by prescribing
  A. Trimethoprim/sulfamethoxazole
  B. Pentamidine isethionate
  C. Amphotericin B
  D. Ketoconazole

4.19 Which of the following should be included on the differential diagnosis list if dysphagia is present in an HIV-positive patient?
A. HIV-related stricture
B. *Candida albicans* esophagitis
C. *Toxoplasma gondii* esophagitis
D. Cryptosporidium esophagitis

4.20 In the HIV-positive individual, a common side effect of ganciclovir is
A. Granulocytopenia
B. Erythrocytosis
C. Hypoglycemia
D. Thrombocytosis

4.21 Appropriate use of CD4 and HIV viral load measurements together includes
A. Monitoring the level of immunosuppression
B. Monitoring the progression of HIV
C. Both
D. Neither

4.22 Which of the following are common clinical manifestations of *M. tuberculosis* in the HIV-infected individual?
A. Lymph node disease
B. Lower lobe involvement in the lung
C. Noncavitary pulmonary involvement
D. Bone marrow involvement
E. All of the above

4.23 Management of *M. tuberculosis* in the HIV-positive individual may include which of the following?
A. Isoniazid and rifampin
B. Ethambutol and pyrazinamide
C. Streptomycin
D. Prolonged and possibly indefinite treatment with antituberculosis drugs
E. All of the above

4.24 Key psychosocial issues that should be addressed in the management of individuals with HIV-1 include
- **A.** Deteriorating health
- **B.** Treatment options
- **C.** Financial insecurity
- **D.** Prospect of death
- **E.** All of the above

4.25 Which of the following has **NOT** been known to transmit HIV-1?
- **A.** Plasma
- **B.** Semen
- **C.** Feces
- **D.** Whole blood

4.26 All of the following are usual modes of HIV-1 transmission **EXCEPT**
- **A.** Casual contact
- **B.** Parenteral exposure to blood or blood products
- **C.** Perinatal transfer from mothers to their infants
- **D.** Sexual contact

4.27 Using the CDC classification system, HIV-positive group C in adults is defined as
- **A.** HIV infection with the development of *P. carinii* pneumonia
- **B.** Initial infection with HIV-1 and no symptoms
- **C.** Initial infection with HIV-1 and associated lymphadenopathy
- **D.** Initial infection with HIV-1 and mononucleosis-like syndrome

4.28 HIV-1 testing is recommended in all of the following populations **EXCEPT**
- **A.** Individuals in mutually monogamous relationships
- **B.** IV drug users
- **C.** Persons who seek treatment for sexually transmitted diseases (STDs)
- **D.** Prostitutes

4.29 All of the following are unique to retroviruses **EXCEPT**
    A. Genetic transfer of information from DNA to RNA
    B. Latency period measured in months to years
    C. Lymphocyte tropism (selective depletion)
    D. Presence of reverse transcriptase

4.30 To obtain the definitive diagnosis of *P. carinii* pneumonia, what diagnostic test is commonly used?
    A. Fiberoptic bronchoscopy with bronchoalveolar lavage
    B. Nonbronchoscopic pulmonary lavage
    C. Open lung biopsy
    D. Ventilation/perfusion lung scan

4.31 All of the following are usually associated with HIV-impaired immunity **EXCEPT**
    A. Allergic rhinitis
    B. Herpes zoster
    C. Herpes genitalis
    D. Tuberculosis

4.32 The most common cause of visual loss in the AIDS patient is
    A. *Cryptococcus neoformans*
    B. Cytomegalovirus
    C. *Mycobacterium avium-intracellulare*
    D. *M. tuberculosis*

4.33 A 31-year-old white man presents with a 7-day history of slurred speech, impaired coordination, and inability to urinate. Social history is remarkable for homosexuality and the use of intravenous drugs. Which of the following should be included in your differential diagnosis?
    A. Primary brain lymphoma
    B. Cryptococcal meningitis
    C. Herpes encephalitis
    D. *T. gondii* encephalitis
    E. All of the above

4.34 A common side effect of aerosolized pentamidine is
    A. Azotemia
    B. Bronchospasm

C. Hypotension
D. Leukopenia

4.35 Infectious dermatologic manifestations of HIV include all of the following **EXCEPT**
A. Human papillomavirus
B. Herpes simplex virus
C. Kaposi's sarcoma
D. Molluscum contagiosum

4.36 In the HIV-1–infected individual, which of the following diagnostic and/or laboratory tests is indicated initially when focal neurologic symptomatology is present?
A. Brain biopsy
B. Computerized tomography/magnetic resonance imaging of the brain
C. Lumbar puncture
D. Pneumoencephalogram

4.37 Regarding herpes zoster in the HIV-infected individual, which of the following is **FALSE?**
A. Clinical zoster occurs as a reactivation of varicella zoster virus and is seen with increased frequency in immuno-compromised patients.
B. Zoster occurs only in patients who have previously been infected with varicella zoster virus (chickenpox).
C. Once the patient is exposed to the virus, it travels from the cutaneous lesions to the sensory neurons and into the dorsal root ganglia, where it remains active.
D. It may involve a single dermatome or multiple dermatomes, and can be recurrent or disseminated.

4.38 Recommended oral care of the HIV-infected patient includes
A. Prophylactic antibiotic coverage for invasive dental procedures in patients with CD4 counts of 800 per cubic millimeter or above
B. Twice-daily rinses with chlorhexidine digluconate
C. Both
D. Neither

4.39 Which of the following diseases is characterized by weight loss and watery diarrhea?
   A. Cryptosporidium
   B. *M. avium* complex
   C. Both
   D. Neither

4.40 Which of the following medications used in the treatment of HIV commonly cause(s) peripheral neuropathy?
   A. Zalcitabine
   B. Didanosine
   C. Zidovudine
   D. A and B only
   E. A, B, and C

HIV/AIDS

Answers and Discussion

4.1 (D) Kaposi's sarcoma (KS) lesions in the AIDS patient may present initially as nonpainful pigmented lesions (usually purple or pink), but may be nonpigmented as well. Many areas may be involved, including the skin and extremities, gastrointestinal tract, oral cavity, and pulmonary parenchyma. Since KS is considered to be an endothelial neoplasm with origins in either capillaries or the lymphatic system, signs of lymphatic obstruction may also be present. (*1, pp 217–218*)

4.2 (E) In the mid-1980s the Centers for Disease Control and Prevention (CDC) developed a surveillance case definition for AIDS in adults and adolescents in order to track the disease. The definition was based on the early observation that patients with AIDS developed certain opportunistic illnesses secondary to a specific defect in a cell-mediated component of the immune system. If no other cause for the cellular dysfunction was present, the diagnosis of 1 of 12 opportunistic illnesses was considered indicative of AIDS. In 1987 the CDC revised this definition to include HIV dementia, HIV wasting syndrome, and other illnesses. More recently, the CDC has expanded the AIDS surveillance definition to include all HIV-infected persons who have fewer than 200 CD4 cells per cubic millimeter or a CD4 cell percentage of total lymphocytes of less than 14. This expansion also includes 3 additional conditions—pulmonary tuberculosis, recurrent pneumonia, and invasive cervical cancer—and retains the 23 conditions in the case definition published in 1987. (*2, pp 1s–15s; 3, pp 1–19*)

4.3 (B) Human immunodeficiency virus (HIV) is the etiologic agent that causes AIDS and has a selective tropism for CD4 cells. Since the CD4 cell is involved in all immune responses, a decrease like the one seen in the HIV infection and AIDS would cause multiple immunologic abnormalities. Hence, B cell abnormalities, decreased parasite killing, and decreased response to soluble antigen would occur. Increased chemotaxis would most likely occur if the immune system remained intact. (*1, p 31*)

4.4 (E) Diseases associated with the pulmonary system are common in individuals infected with HIV. High fevers and shortness of breath are typical symptoms of *P. carinii* and CMV pneumonitis. A dry cough is usually present as well, but not always. Pulmonary tuberculosis and viral pneumonia need to be considered in the differential as well. Tuberculosis is of particular concern because of the growing number of cases that are diagnosed in HIV-infected individuals. (*1, p 67*)

4.5 (D) *P. carinii* pneumonia usually causes a characteristic diffuse interstitial pattern on the chest radiograph. Cytomegalovirus and histoplasmosis can cause this finding as well and should be included on the differential diagnosis list. (*1, p 157*)

4.6 (B) Kaposi's sarcoma is a multifocal neoplasm that can affect any organ in the body. The skin is the most commonly involved organ, and the lesion can present in a variety of forms, colors, shapes, and distribution patterns. Mucous membrane, gastrointestinal, and pulmonary involvement, including involvement of the oral cavity, stomach, colon, small intestine, large bowel, and lungs, may be found in advanced cases. (*1, pp 217–218*)

4.7 (E) The goals of HIV evaluation should include evaluation of the immune system, classification of the HIV infection using the CDC classification system, identification and treatment of infectious and neoplastic complications, institution of approved anti-HIV therapy, and identification of patients who may benefit from experimental therapeutics. (*1, pp 55–57*)

4.8 (E) Once the patient and clinician have decided to initiate antiretroviral therapy, treatment should be aggressive, with the goal of maximal supression of plasma viral load to undetectable levels. In general, any patient with less than 500 CD4 T cells per cubic millimeter or greater than 10,000 (bDNA) or 20,000 (RT-PCR) copies of HIV RNA per milliliter of plasma should be offered therapy. However, the strength of the recommendation for therapy should be based on the readiness of the patient for treatment as well as a consideration of the prognosis for disease-free survival as determined by viral load, CD4 T cell count, and slope of CD4 T cell count decline. (*4, p 5*)

4.9 (D) A thorough history is the most important aspect of the evaluation of a patient infected with HIV. It is essential to identify and distinguish HIV-related conditions from other findings. The focus should be on HIV risk factors, medical history (especially history of STDs), and a comprehensive review of systems. Although it is important to know about childhood allergies, this particular information should not be sought out initially. (*1, pp 57–65*)

4.10 (A) Collectively, pulmonary complications account for the greatest portion of morbidity and mortality in AIDS patients. *P. carinii* is a common AIDS-related infection. Other opportunistic pulmonary infections can be caused by cytomegalovirus, tuberculosis, atypical mycobacteriosis, histoplasmosis, cryptococcosis, and coccidioidomycosis. Neoplasms and lymphoproliferative disorders such as lymphoma, Kaposi's sarcoma, and lymphoid interstitial pneumonitis can also cause pulmonary complications. Vacuolar myelopathy is a degenerative condition in which an open space forms in the spinal cord tissue; it is characterized by a progressive spastic paraparesis and upper motor neuron deficits. Ataxia and hyperreflexia have also been described. (*1, pp 67, 69*)

4.11 (D) Brainstem lymphoma, cryptococcal meningitis, and toxoplasma encephalitis all could occur acutely and have the characteristic signs and symptoms of dizziness, weakness, fevers, and headaches. AIDS dementia complex (ADC) may also have the same signs and symptoms, but usually presents as a slowly progressive disease without focal findings. (*1*, *p 69*)

4.12 (D) Numerous studies have determined that viral load changes precede changes in CD4 counts and are more accurate in determining the relative risk for disease progression as well as the effectiveness of primary therapy. Current consensus is that levels of less than 5,000 to 10,000 copies per milliliter correlate to minimal risk for disease progression, while levels of greater than 30,000 to 100,000 copies per milliliter usually indicate a high risk for disease progression. Higher viral load values over time indicate that primary therapy interventions should be changed or reevaluated and that the risk for opportunistic infections is higher. HIV viral loads are not meant to replace CD4 counts, which are still important in guiding treatment decisions. Their primary value is in guiding and evaluating primary HIV therapy and disease progression. (*1*, *p 255*)

4.13 (D) Trimethoprim (15 to 20 mg/kg/day) and sulfamethoxazole (75 to 100 mg/kg/day), also known as Bactrim or Septra, is the drug of choice when treating *P. carinii* pneumonia. Pentamidine isethionate can also be given if the patient is allergic to Bactrim. Oral atovaquone (750 mg tid) is indicated for second-line treatment for mild to moderate cases of *P. carinii* pneumonia in patients who are intolerant of Bactrim. (*5*, *p 225*)

4.14 (E) Oral candidiasis will respond either to topical therapy, such as nystatin and clotrimazole, or systemic therapy, such as ketoconazole and fluconazole. (*5*, *p 196*)

4.15 (C) Abnormal accumulations of fat in the posterior neck and upper back have been associated with protease inhibitor (PI) treatment. Typically these have occurred after several months of PI administration and have been unresponsive to conservative measures. The adipose nature of the accumulations has been confirmed by imaging procedures or surgical pathology in multiple instances. The exact cause is unknown. (*6, pp 43–44*)

4.16 (D)   Ganciclovir (Cytovene), an acyclovir derivative, has been approved for individuals infected with CMV. The initial dosage is 10 mg/kg/day intravenously divided into two doses for 14 days. Maintenance therapy is required to prevent relapse; recommended doses are 5 mg/kg/day intravenously. Ganciclovir is also available as a capsule for oral administration in a 250-mg strength. Ganciclovir capsules are indicated as an alternative to the intravenous form of ganciclovir for maintenance treatment of CMV. (*5, pp 207–208*)

4.17 (B)   If patients are at risk for HIV infection but their antibody status is unknown, they should be screened for HIV using the enzyme immunoassay (EIA) to detect HIV antibodies. Confirmation of HIV antibodies can be followed up with a Western blot. (*Note:* Seronegative patients must be counseled that testing does not substitute for prevention of HIV; continued high-risk behavior poses a hazard regardless of the frequency of testing.) (*5, p 512*)

4.18 (C)   The primary therapy for cryptococcal meningitis usually employs amphotericin B (0.4 to 0.6 mg/kg/day intravenously for a total of 1.5 to 2.0 g). Fluconazole (400 mg/day) has been approved for the treatment of acute cryptococcal meningitis as well. Fluconazole can be given orally and intravenously, which may shorten hospitalizations and eliminate the use of venous catheters. (*5, pp 202–203*)

4.19 (B)   *C. albicans* and herpes simplex are two agents that may cause dysphagia and esophagitis in an HIV-positive patient. Other possible causes of esophageal pathology include zidovudine therapy, lymphoma, and Kaposi's sarcoma. (*1, p 62*)

4.20 (A)   Individuals infected with HIV and taking ganciclovir may develop granulocytopenia. Granulocytopenia is a commonly encountered cytopenia in HIV infection; besides being caused by drugs (i.e., ganciclovir, retrovir, lamivudine, pyrimethamine, amphotericin B, acyclovir, famcyclovir, trimethoprim/sulfamethoxazole), it may stem from HIV infection alone or may be caused by a myelopathic process in the bone marrow. (*1, p 257*)

4.21 (C) Studies indicate that viral load changes develop early in HIV infection and are accurate in determining the relative risk for disease progression. CD4 cell counts provide a guide to whether the patient is at a negligible, modest, or marked risk for HIV-related opportunistic infection. CD4 counts are also accurate at determining the level of immunosuppression. (*1, pp 252–255*)

4.22 (E) Disseminated disease or limited extrapulmonary tuberculosis (especially in the lymph nodes) occurs in 70% to 80% of HIV-infected patients with tuberculosis. Even when the initial presentation involves the lung, an atypical picture is common. Classical upper lobe apical disease and cavitation are infrequent; chest x-ray films may reveal only adenopathy or middle lobe or lower lobe infiltrates indistinguishable from those produced by other opportunistic infections. Symptoms usually include fever, night sweats, cough, and weight loss, making the diagnosis of tuberculosis difficult to separate from that of other opportunistic diseases. (*1, pp 172–173*)

4.23 (E) Prolonged and possibly indefinite treatment of tuberculosis in the HIV-positive patient is necessary to prevent relapse and further dissemination. Appropriate drugs include isoniazid, rifampin, ethambutol, pyrazinamide, and streptomycin. A common combination of drugs given for active tuberculosis is isoniazid, rifampin, and ethambutol. For multidrug-resistant tuberculosis, five to six drugs are recommended, including isoniazid, rifampin, pyrazinamide, ethambutol, an aminoglycoside (amikacin, streptomycin, kanamycin, capreomycin), and a quinolone (ciprofloxacin, ofloxacin). If a patient presents with resistant strains of TB, an expert should be consulted. (*5, p 223*)

4.24 (E) Patients diagnosed in any group or stage of the HIV infection may develop psychosocial problems apart from physical illness. Fear and uncertainty play a key role in these problems. Patients may face deteriorating health, decisions about treatment, job loss and financial insecurity, loss of emotional support, problems with relationships, changes in lifestyle, and the prospect of death. The clinician must be extremely sensitive to these issues and must be able to identify sources of available support. (*1, pp 77–78*)

4.25 (C) HIV has been isolated from blood and blood products, semen, vaginal secretions, the uterine cervix, saliva, breast milk, tears, urine, cerebrospinal fluid, alveolar fluid, and amniotic fluid. HIV is widely accepted to be transmitted through blood, blood products, and semen. Feces have not been known to transmit the virus, although universal precautions should be adhered to with all body fluids and products. (*1, pp 381–382*)

4.26 (A) HIV is transmitted almost exclusively through sexual contact, through parenteral exposure to blood or blood products, and perinatally from infected mothers to their infants. There have not been any cases linked to casual contact such as hugging or kissing. (*1, pp 17–19*)

4.27 (A) A diagnosis of *P. carinii* pneumonia and other opportunistic infections is indicative of AIDS. (*2, pp 1s–15s; 3, pp 1–19*)

4.28 (A) The U.S. Public Health Service recommends that any individual who has exposure to body fluids or products through sexual activity, parenterally, or perinatally should be counseled and tested for HIV. The Public Health Service also recommends counseling and testing for persons anticipating marriage; for persons who have prolonged diarrhea, lymphadenopathy, fevers, or weight loss; for persons diagnosed with tuberculosis, herpes, or candidiasis; for persons in correctional institutions; and for persons who have had contact with such persons. (*1, pp 301–302*)

4.29 (A) A retrovirus has the ability to transcribe its genetic information from the virion RNA into DNA. This process is aided by the enzyme reverse transcriptase. Research has been directed toward the inhibition of reverse transcriptase in the hope of slowing the replication process of the virus. Nucleoside analogues have been proven to be effective in inhibiting reverse transcriptase. Examples of nucleoside analogues include zidovudine (Retrovir), didanosine (Videx), zalcitabine (Hivid), and stavudine (Zerit). (*1, pp 43–52*)

4.30 **(A)** While nonbronchoscopic pulmonary lavage, open lung biopsy, and ventilation/perfusion lung scan may all be used to diagnose *P. carinii* pneumonia, fiberoptic bronchoscopy with bronchoalveolar lavage remains the most common and most reliable method of diagnosis. The diagnosis of pneumocystis can usually be established by bronchoscopy in over 90% of AIDS patients. (*1, p 157*)

4.31 **(A)** Herpes zoster, herpes genitalis, and tuberculosis can occur with impaired immunity, whereas allergic rhinitis usually does not. A history of recurrent or unusual infections may also suggest impaired immunity. (*1, pp 59–60*)

4.32 **(B)** Cytomegalovirus is by far the most common cause of retinitis and subsequent vision loss in the AIDS patient. Other less common causes of ocular pathology and possible vision loss include toxoplasmosis, herpes simplex, cryptococcus, *C. albicans, M. avium-intracellulare,* and tuberculosis. (*1, p 191*)

4.33 **(E)** Primary brain lymphoma, cryptococcal meningitis, herpes encephalitis, and toxoplasma encephalitis are all possible causes of focal neurologic manifestations and should be included in the differential. (*1, p 69*)

4.34 **(B)** Aerosolized pentamidine has little systemic effect since the drug is not readily absorbed into the bloodstream from the lungs. However, bronchospasms seem to be very common, but easily treated with bronchodilators. (*1, p 267*)

4.35 **(C)** Skin lesions that are most common in HIV-infected patients can be divided into three broad categories: infectious, noninfectious, and neoplastic. Kaposi's sarcoma is a neoplastic lesion. (*1, pp 205–211*)

4.36 (B) Computed tomography (CT) or magnetic resonance imaging (MRI) of the brain is the first diagnostic test that should be done to rule out intracranial lesions. (*1, p 180*)

4.37 (C) Clinical zoster occurs as a reactivation of varicella zoster virus and is seen with increased frequency in immunocompromised patients. Zoster occurs commonly in the elderly but very infrequently in those under 35 years of age. In addition, zoster occurs only in patients who have previously been infected with varicella virus. Upon resolution of the initial infection, the virus travels from the cutaneous lesions to the sensory neurons and into the dorsal root ganglia, where it remains dormant. Herpes zoster may involve a single dermatome or multiple dermatomes and can be recurrent or disseminated. (*1, pp 205–206*)

4.38 (B) Maintenance of immaculate oral hygiene will preserve the dentition and delay oral manifestations, particularly periodontal disease, considerably. Once the CD4 count drops below 200 per cubic millimeter, prophylactic antibiotics are recommended before invasive dental procedures are performed. (*1, p 204*)

4.39 (C) Cryptosporidial infection and *M. avium* are both characterized by weight loss and watery diarrhea. (*1, pp 194–198*)

4.40 (D) Zalcitabine (Hivid) and didanosine (Videx) are commonly associated with the development of peripheral neuropathy. Zidovudine, on the other hand, causes anemia, macrocytosis, nausea, and headaches. (*1, pp 269–271*)

References

1. Muma RD, Lyons BA, Borucki MJ, Pollard RB: *HIV Manual for Health Care Professionals,* Stamford, CT, Appleton & Lange, 1997.

2. Centers for Disease Control: Revision of the CDC surveillance case definition for acquired immunodeficiency syndrome. *MMWR,* 36:1s–15s, 1987.

3. Centers for Disease Control and Prevention: 1993 revised classification system for HIV infection and expanded surveillance case definition for AIDS among adolescents and adults. *MMWR,* 41(RR-17):1–19, 1992.

4. Centers for Disease Control and Prevention: *Guidelines for the Use of Antiretroviral Agents in HIV-Infected Adults and Adolescents,* December 1, 1998.

5. Ungvarski, PJ, Flaskerud JH: *HIV/AIDS: A Guide to Primary Care Management,* Philadelphia, PA, Saunders, 1999.

6. Dube MP, Sattler FR: Metabolic complications of antiretroviral therapies. *AIDS Clin Care* 10, 1998.

5

Pediatrics

Karen S. Stephenson, MS, PA-C

DIRECTIONS (Questions 5.1–5.60): Each of the numbered items or incomplete statements in this chapter is followed by answers or completions of the statement. Select the **one** lettered answer or completion that is **best** in each case.

5.1 All of the following are true about atopic dermatitis **EXCEPT**
  A. The patient usually has a family or personal history of asthma or allergies.
  B. It is marked by severe pruritus.
  C. It is thought to be caused by an imbalance between cytokines.
  D. It usually begins in the newborn period.

5.2 Which of the following factors does **NOT** place a child at higher risk for otitis media?
  A. Age less than 2 years
  B. Attendance at day care
  C. Recurrent tonsillitis
  D. Recurrent antibiotic use

5.3 A 5-year-old is brought to your office because the kindergarten teacher has told the parents that the child is not ready for school. The parents say the teacher has noticed that the child does not handle scissors well or participate appropriately in group activities. All of the following are considered as possibilities for this **EXCEPT**
   A. Delayed language skills
   B. Fine motor dysfunction
   C. Minimal brain dysfunction
   D. Visual loss

5.4 All of the following signs and symptoms point toward the diagnosis of streptococcal pharyngitis **EXCEPT**
   A. Cervical lymphadenopathy
   B. Fever
   C. Headache
   D. Rhinorrhea
   E. Sore throat

5.5 All of the following are expected physical findings in children with allergic rhinitis **EXCEPT**
   A. Clear nasal secretions
   B. Nasal crease
   C. Malocclusion
   D. Red nasal membranes

5.6 Which of the following best describes bacterial conjunctivitis?
   A. Minimal itching, moderate tearing, profuse exudate
   B. Minimal itching, moderate tearing, mucoid exudate
   C. Severe itching, moderate tearing, minimal discharge
   D. None of the above

5.7 Iron-deficiency anemia can be identified by which of the following?
   A. Low MCV and low reticulocyte count
   B. Low MCV and high reticulocyte count
   C. High MCV and low reticulocyte count
   D. High MCV and high reticulocyte count

5.8 Iron-deficiency anemia has also been associated with the development of which of the following?
A. Crohn's disease and ulcerative colitis
B. Impaired cognitive and motor function
C. Hepatic and renal failure
D. Bloody diarrhea and weight loss

5.9 Which of the following describes the results of hemoglobin electrophoresis in someone with sickle cell trait?
A. A_1S
B. SC
C. SS
D. SD

5.10 All of the following may be clinical presentations of acute sickle cell crisis **EXCEPT**
A. Acute chest syndrome
B. Bacterial sepsis
C. Dactylitis
D. Diabetes

5.11 All of the following are true about dactylitis in sickle cell crisis **EXCEPT**
A. It is the most common initial presenting symptom.
B. It is accompanied by marked painful swelling of the hands and feet.
C. It is usually present in younger children.
D. It is usually associated with administration of penicillin.

5.12 All of the following statements describe physiologic jaundice **EXCEPT**
A. It presents on the first day of life.
B. It peaks at less than 14 to 15 on days 3 to 4.
C. The conjugated fraction is less than 2 mg/dL.
D. It persists for no longer than 1 wk.

5.13 ABO incompatibility most commonly occurs with which of the following blood types?
A. Mother type O, baby type B
B. Mother type A, baby type O
C. Mother type AB, baby type O
D. Mother type O, baby type A

5.14 Which of the following describe transient tachypnea of the newborn?
   A. Respiratory distress, shock, poor perfusion, neutropenia
   B. Respiratory distress, barrel-shaped chest, coarse breath sounds
   C. Respiratory distress, perihilar streaking on chest x-ray
   D. Respiratory distress, lack of surfactant

5.15 Which of the following conditions is the most common cause of neonatal seizures?
   A. Drug withdrawal
   B. Hypoglycemia
   C. Hypoxic-ischemic encephalopathy
   D. Intracranial hemorrhage

5.16 All of the following types of infants are at risk for hypoglycemia **EXCEPT**
   A. Infants of diabetic mothers
   B. Infants who are small for gestational age
   C. Infants who have breast milk jaundice
   D. Infants who are stressed at delivery

5.17 All of the following statements about colic are true **EXCEPT**
   A. The infant is described as crying usually in the afternoon.
   B. The infant is otherwise well.
   C. Colic is caused by an allergy to milk.
   D. Colic may occur as result of interaction between infant and caretaker.

5.18 All of the following laboratory values identify infants at low risk for a serious bacterial infection **EXCEPT**
   A. Absolute band count greater than 1500 per cubic millimeter
   B. Stool WBC count less than 10/hpf
   C. Urine WBC count less than 25/hpf
   D. WBC count between 5 and 15×10^3 per cubic millimeter

5.19 Which one of the following symptoms indicates a serious bacterial illness in the febrile infant?
   A. Antibiotic use in the last 7 days
   B. Infant born after 37 wk gestation

C. Normal prenatal course
D. No recent surgery

5.20 Which of the following immunizations has reduced the rates of serious bacterial infections in infants?
A. Hepatitis B
B. *Haemophilus influenzae,* type B
C. MMR
D. Pertussis

5.21 During a well child exam, a 2-mo-old male infant is noticed to have an undescended testis. By what age do most undescended testes enter the scrotal sac normally?
A. 6 mo
B. 12 mo
C. 18 mo
D. 24 mo

5.22 An undescended testis may lose normal morphology and germ cell content by what age?
A. 1 year
B. 2 years
C. 3 years
D. 4 years

5.23 In addition to a hip click, what other physical finding suggests developmental dysplasia of the hip?
A. Dislocation of the patella
B. Limping with ambulation
C. Palpable ischial mass
D. Palpable iliac mass

5.24 Breast-fed babies should receive all of the following while breast-feeding **EXCEPT**
A. Fluoride
B. Iron
C. Vitamin C
D. Vitamin D

5.25 All of the following may indicate tuberculosis in a child **EXCEPT**
  A. Chronic cough
  B. Failure to thrive
  C. Fever
  D. Weight gain

5.26 Which of the following conditions is **NOT** a contraindication for breast-feeding?
  A. Eclampsia
  B. Hemorrhage
  C. Mastitis
  D. Septicemia

5.27 In which of the following infections that can be transmitted by breast milk should breast-feeding be continued if there is no safe alternative?
  A. Cytomegalovirus
  B. Hepatitis B
  C. HIV
  D. Rubella

5.28 The setting sun sign can be noticed in children with which of the following?
  A. Cephalohematoma
  B. Fetal alcohol syndrome
  C. Hydrocephalus
  D. Hypothyroidism

5.29 Infants who are treated for congenital syphilis should be evaluated periodically for resolution of their condition. If the infant is adequately treated, how long should it take for the CSF VDRL to become nonreactive?
  A. 3 mo
  B. 6 mo
  C. 9 mo
  D. 12 mo

5.30 All of the following are true about *Pneumocystis carinii* pneumonia **EXCEPT**
   A. It causes fever, nonproductive cough, and tachypnea.
   B. There are interstitial changes on chest x-ray.
   C. It is treated with amoxicillin.
   D. It is the leading AIDS indicator disease in children.

5.31 Which of the following organisms does **NOT** ordinarily produce blood in the stool?
   A. Campylobacter
   B. Entamoeba
   C. Rotavirus
   D. Salmonella

5.32 If neither blood nor white cells are present in the stool, all of the following are appropriate for the management of diarrhea **EXCEPT**
   A. Rehydration with electrolyte solution
   B. Small amounts of complex carbohydrates (BRAT)
   C. Antimotility agents, such as Imodium
   D. Gradual resumption of lactose products

5.33 All of the following statements about amblyopia are true **EXCEPT**
   A. Amblyopia is suspected when bilateral vision is decreased.
   B. Cataracts may lead to amblyopia.
   C. Children with amblyopia have trouble reading single letters.
   D. Patching of the stronger eye can help correct amblyopia.

5.34 When evaluating a blood level of an anticonvulsant drug, all of the following information is correct **EXCEPT**
   A. The steady state is established at one time the drug's half-life.
   B. Liver and hematopoietic side effects are common with this type of medication.
   C. Blood levels must be correlated with control of seizures.
   D. Frequent changes in dosage may be necessary as a child progresses through adolescence.

5.35 While examining a newborn infant, you notice hypotonia, simian creases, and a heart murmur. Which of the following should you consider most likely as a preliminary diagnosis?
A. Fragile X syndrome
B. Tetralogy of Fallot
C. Trisomy 21
D. Turner syndrome

5.36 Turner syndrome has which genetic abnormality?
A. XY
B. XXY
C. XO
D. YO

5.37 The phenotype for Turner syndrome includes all of the following **EXCEPT**
A. Female appearance
B. Male appearance
C. Short stature
D. Underdeveloped gonads

5.38 Which of the following correctly describes the murmur of ventricular septal defect?
A. Diastolic mitral murmur
B. Aortic systolic murmur
C. Parasternal systolic murmur
D. Pulmonic flow murmur

5.39 A short systolic ejection murmur that is heard best at the left sternal border and without radiation would be which of the following?
A. Aortic stenosis
B. Innocent murmur
C. Pulmonary insufficiency
D. Venous hum

5.40 A 4-year-old is brought to your clinic for fever, sore throat, and rash. The parents report that the rash appeared the night before and is generalized. The rash is more pronounced in skin folds and feels sandpaper-like in texture. You would also expect to find all the following findings **EXCEPT**

A. Pastia sign
B. Circumoral pallor
C. Koplik spots
D. Strawberry tongue

5.41 All of the following are radiologic findings of sinusitis **EXCEPT**
   A. Air-fluid levels
   B. Interstitial markings
   C. Mucosal thickening
   D. Opacification

5.42 All of the following organisms are included among the three most common causes of sinusitis **EXCEPT**
   A. *Borrelia burgdorferi*
   B. *H. influenzae*
   C. *Moraxella catarrhalis*
   D. *Streptococcus pneumoniae*

5.43 Contraindications to induction of emesis in childhood poisoning include all of the following **EXCEPT**
   A. Convulsions
   B. Drowsiness
   C. Presence of gag reflex
   D. Ingestion of drain cleaner

5.44 An adolescent with asthma has recently begun using a peak flow meter to monitor her asthma. She uses a β agonist as needed based on the results of her daily monitoring with the meter. As part of your patient education, you make all of the following recommendations **EXCEPT**
   A. Cough is an important symptom of bronchospasm.
   B. She should begin her inhalant bronchodilator when the meter indicates she is at 20% of her normal peak flow.
   C. She may need to use her inhalant before physical education class and prior to softball games.
   D. If the inhaler is not adequate to control her asthma, steroids or sodium cromolyn may be added.

5.45 How long after birth can the Babinski reflex normally be elicited?
  A. 6 mo
  B. 12 mo
  C. 18 mo
  D. 24 mo

5.46 A retracted eardrum would most likely be associated with which of the following?
  A. Acute otitis media
  B. Cholesteatoma
  C. Perforation
  D. Serous otitis media

5.47 All of the following would allow an infant to be discharged at 24 h **EXCEPT**
  A. Apgar scores of 7 or greater
  B. Blood sugar of 35 mg/dL or greater
  C. Delivery of single vertex infant
  D. Normal physical examination

5.48 Immunologic benefits of breast milk include all of the following **EXCEPT**
  A. Antibodies to poliomyelitis
  B. IgE antibodies to protect mucous membranes
  C. Lactoferrin that protects against *Escherichia coli*
  D. Lipase that inhibits growth of parasites

5.49 All of the following findings help confirm cat scratch disease **EXCEPT**
  A. Intimate exposure to a cat
  B. Inoculation site
  C. Lymphadenopathy
  D. Splenomegaly

5.50 A 2-wk-old is brought to your clinic for a neonatal screen and a checkup. The mother describes a green drainage from the child's left eye that has been present for the last 2 days. All of the following would be in your differential **EXCEPT**
  A. Chlamydia
  B. *Herpes simplex*

C. Staphylococcus
D. Ureaplasma

5.51 If the 2-wk-old in question 5.50 had also presented with tachypnea, was afebrile, and had a staccato cough and rhinorrhea in addition to the conjunctivitis, which of the following would have been the most likely cause?
A. Amoeba
B. Chlamydia
C. Gonorrhea
D. Herpes simplex

5.52 If the infant in question 5.50 had come back for a 2-mo checkup and the mother reported a return of the discharge, all of the following findings would suggest lacrimal duct obstruction **EXCEPT**
A. Discharge on the lashes
B. Eyelids not swollen
C. Red conjunctivae
D. Tearing

5.53 All of the following findings would suggest infantile glaucoma for the infant in question 5.52 **EXCEPT**
A. Cloudy cornea
B. Photophobia
C. Small cornea
D. Tearing

5.54 All of the following statements about scabies are true **EXCEPT**
A. It is caused by mites that burrow under the skin
B. Mites can survive up to 48 h after leaving the host
C. Adolescents have widespread skin involvement
D. 5% permethrin (Elimite) is recommended for infants

5.55 Café-au-lait spots are associated with which one of the following conditions?
A. Halo nevus
B. Mongolian spots
C. Neurofibromatosis
D. Spindle cell nevus

5.56 All of the following are associated with postinfection glomerulonephritis **EXCEPT**
   A. Edema
   B. Hematuria
   C. Hypotension
   D. Renal insufficiency

5.57 Urinalysis demonstrates all of the following in postinfection glomerulonephritis **EXCEPT**
   A. Proteinuria
   B. Red blood cells
   C. Red blood cell casts
   D. White blood cell casts

5.58 A 3-year-old girl is brought to your office because she has had pain with urination. In addition to cystitis, all but which one of the following should be considered as part of the differential diagnosis?
   A. Anal fistula
   B. Pinworm infestation
   C. Vulvitis from *Candida albicans*
   D. Vulvitis from bubble bath

5.59 Which of the following would be the most likely organism to cause urinary tract infections in children?
   A. Chlamydia
   B. *E. coli*
   C. Klebsiella
   D. Proteus

5.60 When hypospadias is discovered in a newborn male infant, all of the following should be ruled out as part of the examination **EXCEPT**
   A. Ambiguous genitalia
   B. Atresia of the rectum
   C. Inguinal hernias
   D. Undescended testes

Pediatrics

Answers and Discussion

5.1 (D) Atopic dermatitis usually develops between 2 and 6 mo of age in 60% of children who develop this skin condition. (*1, pp 394–395*)

5.2 (C) Recurrent otitis media rather than recurrent tonsillitis places children at greater risk of another ear infection. (*2, p 456*)

5.3 (D) Major visual problems are usually detected in infancy, and any visual problems present in this situation result from a neurologic cause rather than an ophthalmologic one. Children should receive a complete workup including auditory testing, intellectual functioning, and neurologic function. Minimal brain dysfunction is the most common cause of school unreadiness. (*3, p 151*)

5.4 (D) Rhinorrhea, cough, and conjunctivitis point toward a viral cause. Exudate may be present in pharyngitis with both bacterial and viral etiologies. The diagnosis should be confirmed by rapid strep testing or throat culture. (*4, pp 482–484*)

5.5 (D) Nasal membranes in allergy are usually pale rather than red and contain many eosinophils. (*5, p 181*)

5.6 (A)   B describes viral conjunctivitis and C describes allergic conjunctivitis. Bacterial causes should be established by culture and may be treated with broad-spectrum antibiotic drops. There is no agent for viruses, but sulfonamide drops may be given to protect against secondary infections, and allergic conjunctivitis can be treated with vasoconstrictive agents, antihistamines, or, for short periods of time, topical corticosteroids. (*6, pp 431–432*)

5.7 (A)   The reticulocyte count may be elevated in iron-deficiency anemia, however. (*7, pp 819–820*)

5.8 (B)   Children with iron-deficiency anemia may be irritable and display delayed motor and cognitive function. (*7, p 823*)

5.9 (A)   This is expected hemoglobin for someone with sickle cell trait, i.e., the individual is a carrier for the sickle gene, and SS is the pattern for sickle cell disease. The other two are hemoglobins that combine with the sickled hemoglobin. (*7, pp 832, 834*)

5.10 (D)   All of the others are signs of crisis. Acute chest syndrome presents with fever, pleuritic chest pain, pulmonary infiltrates, and hypoxemia. See question 5.11 for dactylitis. (*7, p 832*)

5.11 (D)   Dactylitis is not associated with penicillin. (*7, p 832*)

5.12 (A)   Jaundice that appears on the first day is not physiologic and warrants a workup. (*8, p 37*)

5.13 (D)   Type O is the most common blood type, and type A is the second most common; ABO incompatibility can also occur with babies having type B blood, but it is less common. The mother's IgG anti-A or anti-B crosses the placenta and destroys the baby's red blood cells. (*8, p 39*)

5.14 (C)   A describes congenital pneumonia, B describes meconium aspiration syndrome, and D describes hyaline membrane disease. Transient tachypnea usually resolves in 12 to 24 h and is thought to result from delayed resorption of fetal lung fluid. (*8, p 33*)

5.15 (C) Signs of hypoxic-ischemic encephalopathy include decreased level of consciousness, seizures, apnea, jitteriness, hypotonia, and brainstem signs. (*8, p 62*)

5.16 (C) Infants who might have jaundice and hypoglycemia are more likely to have erythroblastosis (Rh-negative blood type). (*8, p 54*)

5.17 (C) Colic has long been thought to have some gastrointestinal cause, though none has ever been proven. Wessel has defined colic as occurring in a well child who cries for more than 3 h/day for more than 3 days/wk and for more than 3 wk. Though changing the formula is a common treatment for colic, support for the parents and techniques for dealing with colic (taking the baby for a car ride, for example) are more appropriate. (*9, p 197*)

5.18 (A) For infants 3 mo of age or less, the absolute band count should be less than 1500 per cubic millimeter. These lab values can be used along with history and physical findings to identify children at low risk. (*10, p 118*)

5.19 (A) Recent antibiotic use places the infant at greater risk of serious bacterial illness. (*10, p 101*)

5.20 (B) The *H. influenzae* type B immunization has reduced the rate of serious infections. (*10, p 119*)

5.21 (B) By 12 mo of age, 80% of testes that were undescended at birth have entered the scrotal sac; most undescended testes are unilateral. (*11, p 642*)

5.22 (B) Biopsy specimens demonstrate the loss of normal testicular tissue by 2 years of age. Undescended testes are also 40 times more likely than descended testes to become malignant, with tumors usually developing between 25 and 30 years of age. (*11, p 643*)

5.23 (B) Limping may occur in the walking child; when both hips are dislocated, the child may waddle. There may also be lax hamstrings that allow full extension of the knee when the hip is in flexion and telescoping in which the hip can be pulled back and forth at 90° of flexion. (*12, p 688*)

5.24 (C) Vitamin C supplementation is generally not needed by the breast-fed infant. (*13, pp 484–486*)

5.25 (D) Another symptom of tuberculosis may be anorexia. Most children with tuberculosis are without symptoms, however. (*14, p 523*)

5.26 (C) Mastitis that has been treated is not a contraindication to continued breast-feeding. (*13, pp 28, 230*)

5.27 (C) In countries in which there is refrigeration available, mothers who are HIV+ should not breast-feed. If there is no refrigeration, then breast milk should be continued. (*13, p 151*)

5.28 (C) Collecting cerebrospinal fluid leads to increased CNS pressure. A bulging fontanelle may also be noted. (*15, p 656*)

5.29 (B) If the CSF remains positive past 6 mo, the infant with congenital syphilis should be retreated. Infants with congenital syphilis should be followed closely for neurologic or ophthalmologic complications of the disease. (*16, p 195*)

5.30 (D) PCP is usually treated with sulfa drugs or pentamidine. (*16, pp 182–183*)

5.31 (C) Rotavirus usually causes vomiting and diarrhea during the winter season, with associated respiratory symptoms and low-grade fever. It ordinarily does not produce blood in the stool, but may do so in infants. Rotavirus is the most common cause of diarrhea in children less than 2 years of age in developed countries. The organism can be identified by assay of the stool. (*17, pp 625–626*)

5.32 (C) The emphasis of treatment for diarrhea should be on maintaining the child's hydration. The villi of the small intestine take several days to grow back and the stool will gradually become firm again. Imodium is contraindicated in children less than 2 years of age and in children who have blood in the stool and fever. (*17, pp 625–626*)

5.33 (C) Children with amblyopia can read single letters more easily than a row of letters. This inability to read rows of letters is referred to as the crowding phenomenon. (*18, pp 555–556*)

5.34 (A) Most steady states are not established until two to three times the half-life of the drug. Adolescents with seizure disorders are at risk for not taking their medication because of peer pressure or self-esteem issues. As these children grow, rapid changes in dosages because of weight gain may be necessary to maintain control of seizures. (*19, pp 731–732*)

5.35 (C) Trisomy 21 is the most common chromosomal syndrome. Other findings include epicanthal folds, protruding tongue, beaded irises, high-arched palate, short neck, and short, broad hands. (*20, p 328*)

5.36 (C) Turner syndrome results from a loss of all or part of one of the sex chromosomes. (*20, p 330*)

5.37 (B) The appearance of the patient with Turner syndrome is that of a female. (*20, p 330*)

5.38 (C) This is the classic description of ventricular septal defect, the most common cause of congenital heart disease. (*21, p 1167*)

5.39 (B) Thirty percent of children have this murmur, and it is accentuated by fever, excitement, or exercise. A ventricular septal defect can be heard in this same area, but it sounds loud, harsh, or blowing, and is frequently accompanied by a thrill. (*21, p 1132*)

5.40 (C) The condition is scarlet fever. Koplik spots appear on the buccal mucosa across from the molars in people with measles. The Pastia sign refers to a petechial rash in the antecubital area. Throat culture or rapid streptococcal screening will usually identify the cause. Penicillin is the treatment of choice. (*22, p 700*)

5.41 (B) Interstitial markings are usually a chest x-ray finding in viral or mycoplasma infection. Air-fluid levels on sinus films are uncommon in children less than 5 years of age. Mucosal thickening of 4 mm or greater in children or 5 mm or greater in adults is very common in sinusitis. (*23, p 311*)

5.42 (A) Borrelia is the spirochete that causes Lyme disease; the other three bacteria commonly cause acute sinusitis. (*23, p 311*)

5.43 (C) An intact gag reflex can help protect against aspiration. Convulsions and drowsiness also increase the risk of aspiration. Drain cleaners, as well as other bases, acids, and some hydrocarbons, should not be removed by emesis. Poison control centers should also be consulted. (*24, p 320*)

5.44 (B) The dosage or frequency of asthma medication should be increased when the peak flow meter reveals the peak flow reading to be 70% of best peak flow. Coughing may be a more sensitive indicator of bronchospasm than waiting until wheezing begins. If the peak flow reading is 50% or less, medical attention should be sought. (*25, p 186*)

5.45 (D) Most newborns (90%) have a flexion response to stimulation, but the Babinski reflex may be present for as long as 24 mo. A Babinski response that is present later than expected warrants a workup for central nervous system disease. (*15, pp 627, 633*)

5.46 (D) Serous otitis media usually results from viral upper respiratory infection or allergic rhinitis, and both air and fluid are present in the middle ear space. When viewed, the bony anatomy is prominent and amber fluid may be seen. (*26, p 217*)

5.47 (B) Blood sugars need to be maintained at 45 mg/dL or greater. Both small- and large-for-gestational-age babies may have blood sugar regulation problems. Small-for-gestational-age babies do not have fat stores to mobilize, and large-for-gestational-age babies have been producing large amounts of insulin to deal with hyperglycemia from their mothers. (*8, p 54*)

5.48 (B) IgA protects mucous membranes and is present in human milk. (*13, pp 138–139*)

5.49 (D) Splenomegaly is usually not a part of cat scratch disease. The cat is usually immature. The inoculation site is usually a pustule that develops adjacent to the lymphadenopathy. The inoculation lesion progresses through the same stages that a chicken pox lesion does. (*27, pp 758–760*)

5.50 (D) Other causes of ophthalmia neonatorum include gonorrhea, pneumococcus, or silver nitrate instillation. Chlamydia is the most common cause, and 50% of infants exposed to chlamydia by their mothers develop this eye infection. (*6, p 433*)

5.51 (B) The infection is treated with oral erythromycin. (*28, p 736*)

5.52 (C) Red conjunctivae and discharge suggest conjunctivitis. Some children with obstruction may have secondary conjunctivitis. (*29, pp 379–380*)

5.53 (C) The cornea is enlarged rather than shrunken. After age 2 years, the cornea does not enlarge even with increased intraocular pressure. (*29, pp 380–381*)

5.54 (C) Adolescents and older children tend to have scabies in interdigital spaces, spaces of flexure, the buttocks, and around the areolas. Infants are more likely to have widespread involvement. (*30, pp 275–276*)

5.55 (C) Five or more café-au-lait spots usually occur with neurofibromatosis, and the axillae should be checked for freckling. (*31, p 273*)

5.56 (C) Hypertension rather than hypotension is usually associated with postinfection glomerulonephritis. (*32, pp 1329–1331*)

5.57 (D) White blood cell casts are caused by a primary infection in the kidney, whereas the damage to the kidney in nephritis is caused by antibody-antigen complexes from skin or throat streptococcal infection that are deposited in the kidney. (*32, pp 1329–1331*)

5.58 (A) Pinworms can be observed in the perianal area at night. Vulvitis from yeast infections or bubble bath irritation may mimic cystitis. In girls, perineal hygiene, including wiping after urinating, should be addressed. Many small children wipe from back to front instead of front to back. (*33, p 1362*)

5.59 (B) *E. coli* is the most common cause of UTIs overall, but klebsiella and proteus can also cause infection. Chlamydia would not be an expected organism. (*33, p 1360*)

5.60 (B) Hypospadias is associated with other genital anomalies. All patients with hypospadias and undescended testes should have a karyotype. Patients with hypospadias should not be circumcised, so that the foreskin can be used to repair the urethra. (*33, p 1377*)

References

1. Paller A: Atopic dermatitis. In: Dershewitz RA (ed): *Ambulatory Pediatric Care*, 3/e, Philadelphia, Lippincott-Raven, 1999.

2. Macknin M: Acute otitis media. In: Dershewitz RA (ed): *Ambulatory Pediatric Care*, 3/e, Philadelphia, Lippincott-Raven, 1999.

3. Shapiro BK: School readiness. In: Dershewitz RA (ed): *Ambulatory Pediatric Care*, 3/e, Philadelphia, Lippincott-Raven, 1999.

4. Niederman LG, Marcinak JF: Sore throat. In: Dershewitz RA (ed): *Ambulatory Pediatric Care*, 3/e, Philadelphia, Lippincott-Raven, 1999.

5. Bailit IW: Allergic rhinitis. In: Dershewitz RA (ed): *Ambulatory Pediatric Care*, 2/e, Philadelphia, Lippincott, 1993.

6. Ellis PP: Eye. In: Hay WW (ed): *Current Pediatric Diagnosis and Treatment*, 12/e, Norwalk, CT, Appleton & Lange, 1995.

7. Lane PA, Nuss R, Ambruso, DR: Hematologic disorders. In: Hay WW (ed): *Current Pediatric Diagnosis and Treatment*, 12/e, Norwalk, CT, Appleton & Lange, 1995.

8. Rosenberg AA, Thilo EH: The newborn infant. In: Hay WW (ed): *Current Pediatric Diagnosis and Treatment*, 12/e, Norwalk, CT, Appleton & Lange, 1995.

9. Goldson E: Behavioral disorders and developmental variations. In: Hay WW (ed): *Current Pediatric Diagnosis and Treatment*, 12/e, Norwalk, CT, Appleton & Lange, 1995.

10. Slater M, Krug SE: Evaluation of the infant with fever without source: An evidence-based approach. *Emerg Med Clin North Am* 17(1):97–126, 1999.

11. Foglia RP: Undescended testes. In: Dershewitz RA (ed): *Ambulatory Pediatric Care,* 3/e, Philadelphia, Lippincott-Raven, 1999.

12. Brown LM: Developmental dysplasia of the hip (congenital dislocation of the hip). In: Dershewitz RA (ed): *Ambulatory Pediatric Care,* 3/e, Philadelphia, Lippincott-Raven, 1999.

13. Curran JS, Barness LA: Nutrition. In: Behrman RE, Kliegman RM, Jenson HB (eds): *Nelson Textbook of Pediatrics,* 16/e, Philadelphia, Saunders, 2000.

14. Larsen GL et al: Respiratory tract and mediastinum. In: Hay WW (ed): *Current Pediatric Diagnosis and Treatment,* 12/e, Norwalk, CT, Appleton & Lange, 1995.

15. Hoekelman RA: The physical examination of infants and children. In: Bickley LS (ed): *Bates' Guide to Physical Examination and History Taking,* 7/e, Philadelphia, Lippincott, 1999.

16. Stephenson KS: Pediatric HIV infection. In: Muma RD et al (eds): *HIV Manual for Health Care Professionals.* Norwalk, CT, Appleton & Lange, 1994.

17. Sondheimer JM, Silverman A: Gastrointestinal tract. In: Hay WW (ed): *Current Pediatric Diagnosis and Treatment,* 12/e, Norwalk, CT, Appleton & Lange, 1995.

18. Zwaan J: Amblyopia. In: Dershewitz RA (ed): *Ambulatory Pediatric Care,* 3/e, Philadelphia, Lippincott-Raven, 1999.

19. Moe PG, Seay AR: Neurologic and muscular disorders. In: Hay WW (ed): *Current Pediatric Diagnosis and Treatment,* 12/e, Norwalk, CT, Appleton & Lange, 1995.

20. Hall JG: Chromosomal clinical abnormalities. In: Behrman RE, Kliegman RM, Jenson HB (eds): *Nelson Textbook of Pediatrics,* 16/e, Philadelphia, Saunders, 2000.

21. Pruitt AW: The cardiovascular system. In: Behrman RE et al (eds): *Nelson Textbook of Pediatrics,* 14/e, Philadelphia, Saunders, 1992.

22. Kliegman RM, Feigin RD: Streptococcal infections. In: Behrman RE et al (eds): *Nelson Textbook of Pediatrics,* 14/e, Philadelphia, Saunders, 1992.

23. Wald ER: Sinusitis. In: Dershewitz RA (ed): *Ambulatory Pediatric Care,* 2/e, Philadelphia, Lippincott, 1993.

24. Dart RC, Rumack BH: Poisoning. In: Hay WW (ed): *Current Pediatric Diagnosis and Treatment,* 12/e, Norwalk, CT, Appleton & Lange, 1995.

25. Lapey A: Asthma. In: Dershewitz RA (ed): *Ambulatory Pediatric Care,* 2/e, Philadelphia, Lippincott, 1993.

26. Bates B: *A Guide to Physical Examination and History Taking,* 5/e, Philadelphia, Lippincott, 1991.

27. Carthers HA: Cat-scratch disease. In: Dershewitz RA (ed): *Ambulatory Pediatric Care,* 2/e, Philadelphia, Lippincott, 1993.

28. Dashefsky B: Sexually transmitted disease. In: Dershewitz RA (ed): *Ambulatory Pediatric Care,* 2/e, Philadelphia, Lippincott, 1993.

29. Boger WP: Tearing. In: Dershewitz RA (ed): *Ambulatory Pediatric Care,* 2/e, Philadelphia, Lippincott, 1993.

30. Paller A: Insect bites and infestations. In: Dershewitz RA (ed): *Ambulatory Pediatric Care,* 2/e, Philadelphia, Lippincott, 1993.

31. Paller A: Epidermal tumors. In: Dershewitz RA (ed): *Ambulatory Pediatric Care,* 2/e, Philadelphia, Lippincott, 1993.

32. Bergstein JM: Nephrologic diseases. In: Behrman RE et al (eds): *Nelson Textbook of Pediatrics,* 14/e, Philadelphia, Saunders, 1992.

33. Gonzales R: Urologic disorders in infants and children. In: Behrman RE et al (eds): *Nelson Textbook of Pediatrics,* 14/e, Philadelphia, Saunders, 1992.

6

Orthopedics

Albert F. Simon, MEd, PA-C

DIRECTIONS (Questions 6.1–6.40): Each of the numbered items or incomplete statements is this chapter is followed by answers or completions of the statement. Select the **one** lettered answer or completion that is **best** in each case.

6.1 A 59-year-old woman presents with painful joints of several months duration. Examination of fluid from a joint reveals
Clarity: transparent
Color: yellow
WBCs: 300
PMNs: 15% of sample
Glucose: equal to serum

This is most consistent with
    A. Septic arthritis
    B. Normal joint aspirate
    C. Acute gout
    D. Osteoarthritis
    E. Rheumatoid arthritis

6.2 Which of the following is **NOT** true of osteoarthritis?
  A. Recreational running does not increase incidence.
  B. A key component is inflammation of symmetrical joints.
  C. It is characterized by articular stiffness that lasts less than 15 min.
  D. Obesity is a risk factor for development.
  E. It is the most common form of joint disease.

6.3 Effective treatment of gout includes
  A. Starting the patient on loop diuretics
  B. Placing the patient on a high-protein diet and moderating alcohol intake
  C. Using steroids in doses of 40 mg/day as first-line treatment to quell inflammation of acute attacks
  D. Treating hyperuricemia immediately with uricosuric agents
  E. Placing the patient with an acute attack on bed rest for about 24 h after the attack has subsided

6.4 Which of the following statements is true about gout?
  A. It has equal prevalence in men and women.
  B. Its highest incidence is in Hispanic populations.
  C. Onset in women is usually postmenopausal.
  D. Tophi typically develop in the ears, hands, and other tissues shortly after the first attack.
  E. Crystals appear rhomboid under light-microscopy.

6.5 Which of the following diseases has been demonstrated to reduce life expectancy?
  A. Rheumatoid arthritis
  B. Osteoarthritis
  C. Gout
  D. Degenerative joint disease
  E. Chondrocalcinosis

6.6 Agents that inhibit COX-2 (proinflammatory) enzyme systems when used to treat pain from rheumatoid arthritis have been found
  A. To be in the category of disease-modifying antirheumatoid drugs
  B. To be safer than other NSAIDs in treating arthritis

C. Not to cause liver enzyme elevation like other NSAIDs
D. To be more effective than other NSAIDs in treating arthritis
E. To decrease extraarticular manifestations of the disease

6.7 Which of the following is considered the drug of choice for patients with rheumatoid arthritis?
A. Methotrexate
B. Corticosteroids
C. Hydroxychloroquine
D. Gold salts
E. Sulfasalazine

6.8 A 50-year-old man who is employed as a fire fighter presents with complaints of right arm pain × 1 mo. The pain is aggravated by sneezing, coughing, and raising the arm up to the shoulder. Exam reveals a decrease in the biceps reflex on the right side. Based on the history and physical findings, what is the likely diagnosis?
A. Cervical spondylosis
B. Cervical strain
C. Thoracic outlet syndrome
D. Chondrocalcinosis
E. Herniated cervical nucleus pulposus

6.9 What is the appropriate treatment of the patient in question 6.8 at this time?
A. Referral to surgery
B. Bed rest and NSAIDs
C. Epidural steroid injection
D. Bracing
E. Steroid injection into the facet joint

6.10 A 53-year-old man presents with complaints of back pain that he attributes to "lumbago." History reveals that this patient has a 30-pack-year smoking history. He has been trying to lose some weight and has done better than expected, losing 20 lb in the last 6 wk. He denies morning stiffness but complains of "sore joints" in his hands and wrists made worse with activity. What diagnostic concern does this history raise?

    A. Rheumatoid arthritis
    B. Prostate cancer with metastasis
    C. Reiter syndrome
    D. HNP of the lumbar spine
    E. Ankylosing spondylitis

6.11 Which is true of the musculoskeletal system?

    A. Peak bone mass is reached at about 25 years of age for men and 40 years of age for women.
    B. Bone growth is completed at about age 20 in both genders.
    C. Long bones increase in length by growth from ossification centers in calcified cartilage.
    D. Bones are stronger than ligaments until adolescence.
    E. During late pregnancy, the degree of normal lordosis decreases to shift the center of gravity over the lower extremity.

6.12 Which of the following patients is **LEAST** likely to develop osteoporosis? (All are post-menopausal.)

    A. A 62-year-old African American woman with hypertension
    B. A 63-year-old Caucasian woman in good health
    C. A 62-year-old Asian woman with a history of HPV infection
    D. A 61-year-old Native American woman in good health

6.13 A 21-year-old patient arrives in the emergency department with a leg injury secondary to an MVA. X-ray examination reveals a fracture of the tibia. You note that there is a large free-floating piece of bone between well-defined fracture lines superior and inferior to it. This would be most correctly described as a _____ fracture.

A. Segmental
B. Comminuted
C. Spiral
D. Torus
E. Transverse

6.14 A 5-year-old child suffers an injury to her lower extremity when she falls approximately 8 ft and lands in the standing position. What type of Salter fracture is most likely?
A. Type I
B. Type II
C. Type III
D. Type IV
E. Type V

6.15 A 12-year-old boy sustains a nondisplaced fracture of the ulna. Which of the following splints would be appropriate for initial immobilization?
A. Long arm gutter
B. Short arm gutter
C. Cock-up
D. Sugar tong
E. Thumb spica

6.16 Which nerve is tested by having the patient spread and push the fingers together against resistance?
A. Median
B. Ulnar
C. Radial
D. Digital

6.17 A 4-year-old child is brought to the office due to an arm injury. An impatient baby-sitter pulled on the hand of the child and now the child refrains from using that arm. The patient is in no apparent distress. Choose the correct statement concerning this condition.
A. This injury is most common in 7- to 10-year-olds.
B. Treatment involves extending the elbow.
C. Frequently the neurovascular exam reveals radial artery compromise.
D. The injured arm is usually held in pronation and flexion.

6.18 A 10-year-old boy has been treated for a supracondylar fracture of the right arm. He now presents with pain and refrains from opening his right hand. All of the following findings would be expected, **EXCEPT**
  A. Absent radial pulse
  B. Pain on passive extension of fingers
  C. Isolated radial nerve paralysis
  D. Pallor of the extremity
  E. Forearm tenderness

6.19 A 50-year-old man presents with acute pain in the upper right arm and shoulder. The patient relates a history of "snapping" over the area for the last 3 wk. On examination, you note that (1) flexion of the elbow elicits pain; (2) there is local tenderness of the biceps and anterior shoulder; and (3) there is an egg-shaped swelling in the biceps on the affected arm. These findings are most consistent with
  A. Bicipital tendinitis
  B. Osteochondral fracture
  C. Biceps rupture
  D. Impingement syndrome
  E. Rotator cuff damage

6.20 The single best test of radial nerve friction is the ability to
  A. Make an OK sign with the fingers
  B. Abduct the index finger
  C. Close and open the fingers against resistance
  D. Make a "steeple" with the index fingers
  E. Extend the wrist and fingers against resistance

6.21 Which bone of the wrist is most commonly fractured?
  A. Distal radius
  B. Distal ulna
  C. Navicular
  D. Pisiform
  E. Lunate

6.22 A patient falls on the outstretched hand while walking and presents with left wrist pain. Which of the following is true concerning the injury?

A. Triquetrum fractures present with avascular necrosis as often as do navicular fractures.
B. Navicular fractures are easily diagnosed on plain radiographs.
C. A single view of the wrist would be adequate to evaluate this injury.
D. Navicular fractures are the most common carpal fractures.
E. Pain on the ulnar aspect of the wrist raises suspicion of a navicular fracture regardless of how the x-ray looks.

6.23 An 82-year-old woman presents to the emergency department after a fall in her home. She is not able to walk or bear weight on her right leg. There is marked pain in her right hip. Exam reveals some shortening of the right limb and some external rotation. What is the likely diagnosis?
A. Femoral shaft fracture
B. Femoral neck fracture
C. Intertrochanteric fracture
D. Anterior dislocation
E. Femoral head fracture

6.24 A 24-year-old patient presents after a skiing injury to the left knee the night before. Choose the correct statement concerning knee injuries.
A. History of painful locking points toward cruciate tear.
B. The medial meniscus is more likely to be torn than the lateral.
C. Think of posterior cruciate tears if the patient hears a "pop" with the injury.
D. Tests like the McMurray test accurately identify a torn meniscus over 90% of the time.
E. The anterior drawer test is most sensitive in diagnosing anterior cruciate tears.

6.25 Which is not part of the initial treatment for a single torn ligament in the knee?
A. Ice
B. Knee immobilization
C. NSAIDs
D. Referral for surgical repair
E. Elevation

6.26 The recommended treatment of shin splints is
   A. Ultrasound therapy
   B. Cessation of offending activity for several weeks
   C. Rest × 3 days followed by application of heat
   D. NSAIDs
   E. Application of brace during activity

6.27 The preferred initial treatment for a wrist ganglion is
   A. Forceful compression with a book
   B. Injection with steroids
   C. Aspiration and chemical cauterization
   D. NSAIDs
   E. Surgical excision

6.28 A 30-year-old man presents with left shoulder pain. There is no history of acute injury, but the patient participates in several sports. Examination reveals tenderness approximately 2 cm below the tip of the acromion. There is also pain in the left shoulder as the patient supinates against resistance. What is the most likely diagnosis?
   A. Rotator cuff tear
   B. Adhesive capsulitis
   C. Rotator cuff tendinitis
   D. First-degree sprain of AC joint
   E. Bicipital tendinitis

6.29 A 17-year-old high school cheerleader presents with difficulty walking and ankle pain after landing on her dorsiflexed foot during practice. She states it felt like someone kicked her in the back of the leg. Choose the true statement concerning this case.
   A. Standard ankle x-rays are just as helpful in the diagnosis as MRI.
   B. This patient will probably not be able to walk on her toes.
   C. There will be weak or absent plantar extension.
   D. Initial treatment is surgery.
   E. This condition often occurs with repetitive hill running.

6.30 A patient with adhesive capsulitis
   A. Complains of decreased ROM of the shoulder
   B. Is likely to be elderly

C. Often is unable to raise the arms above the head
D. Demonstrates a decrease in passive ROM
E. All of the above

6.31 Which is true of mechanical low back pain?
A. Symptoms are usually aggravated with rest.
B. Less than 5% of patients develop chronic low back syndrome.
C. Traction usually provides significant relief.
D. Narcotics will provide relief if used in therapeutic doses for more than 3 wk.
E. Treatment with bed rest should be continued for at least 7 days.

6.32 Which statement is true concerning spinal tumors?
A. Spinal tumors are common bone tumors.
B. Pain made worse with activity suggests a tumor.
C. Multiple myeloma is the most common malignant primary bone tumor.
D. Although common, tumors in the vertebral body are usually benign.
E. Most spinal tumors in people under 21 years of age are malignant.

6.33 In the evaluation of the patient with LBP, x-rays should be ordered routinely **EXCEPT**
A. For suspected fracture
B. For suspected infection of the spine
C. To identify degenerative changes
D. For suspected developmental abnormality
E. For medicolegal documentation for worker's compensation

6.34 Which of the following is the most common cause of low back pain in children and adolescents?
A. Scoliosis
B. Herniated lumbar disc
C. Spondylolysis
D. Spondyloesthesis
E. Spinal stenosis

6.35 Painless, hard nodules located at the PIP joints on the hand of a 58-year-old laborer are probably associated with
    A. Rheumatoid arthritis
    B. Reiter syndrome
    C. Osteoarthritis
    D. Tophaceous gout
    E. Ankylosing spondylitis

6.36 A 32-year-old female patient with a positive Tinel test should also demonstrate
    A. Numbness of the 4th and 5th digits
    B. Decreased ulnar nerve conduction velocities
    C. A positive Finkelstein test
    D. Thenar atrophy
    E. Weakness of wrist

6.37 Which bursa is particularly susceptible to developing septic bursitis?
    A. Ischial
    B. Subacromial
    C. Olecranon
    D. Trochanteric
    E. Gastrocnemio-semimembranous

6.38 Which of the following steroid preparations would be best suited for injection into deeper tissues?
    A. Triamcinolone hexacetonide
    B. Prednisolone sodium phosphate
    C. Prednisolone tebutate
    D. Prednisolone hydrochloride

6.39 Which is true of fibromyalgia syndrome?
    A. It most commonly affects older men.
    B. Chronic pain must be present for at least 6 mo for diagnosis.
    C. CP inflammation is prominent.
    D. The key to treatment is administration of antidepressants and muscle relaxants concomitantly.
    E. It usually responds well to amitriptyline given at bedtime.

6.40 The most commonly injured ligament in the knee is the
 A. Anterior cruciate
 B. Posterior cruciate
 C. Lateral collateral ligament
 D. Medial collateral ligament
 E. Medial meniscus

Orthopedics

Answers and Discussion

6.1 (D) The low WBC count, PMNs less than 25%, and glucose levels equal to the serum point toward a noninflammatory arthritis like osteoarthritis. (*1, p 808*)

6.2 (B) Inflammation is not usually present in osteoarthritis; when it does occur, it affects the IP joints acutely. (*1, p 808*)

6.3 (E) Early ambulation of the patient with acute gout may cause a flare-up. Bed rest for about 24 h after the acute attack subsides is advisable. (*1, p 812*)

6.4 (C) The frequency of gout in women is much lower than in men, and its onset in women is usually much later than in men. It often begins after menopause. (*1, p 810*)

6.5 (A) Having many articular and extraarticular manifestations, rheumatoid arthritis has been shown to decrease life expectancy. (*1, p 832*)

6.6 (B) COX 2 inhibitors like celecoxib (Celebrex) have been shown to cause fewer GI side effects than other NSAIDs when used to treat arthritis. (*1, p 829*)

6.7 (A) Of the agents listed, methotrexate is considered by many to be the drug of choice for treatment of rheumatoid arthritis. The second-line agent is sulfasalazine. (*1, pp 830–831*)

6.8 (E) Patients with cervical herniated nucleus pulposus often present with upper extremity pain that increases with increased intraabdominal pressure and arm motion. (*1, p 815*)

6.9 (B) Initial treatment of cervical HNP includes conservative measures like intermittent cervical traction, rest, and NSAIDs. (*1, p 815*)

6.10 (B) Age beyond 50 years, smoking, and weight loss are all risk factors for metastatic cancer to the vertebral column. (*1, p 817*)

6.11 (B) Ossification occurs at specific time intervals in the skeleton. Growth is completed in both sexes at around 20 years of age. (*2, p 700*)

6.12 (A) African American women have bone densities that resemble those of white men, making osteoporosis less likely. (*2, p 701*)

6.13 (A) A segmental fracture is present when a free-floating piece of bone is bordered by two well-defined fracture lines. (*3, p 1743*)

6.14 (E) A Salter type V fracture should be suspected when a great degree of axial loading has been applied to the bone. (*3, p 1745*)

6.15 (D) The sugar tong splint is appropriate for fractures of the wrist and distal forearm. (*3, p 1749*)

6.16 (B) The ulnar nerve innervates the motor function of the hypothenar interossei and the ulnar two lumbricals. (*3, p 1754*)

6.17 (B) Treatment of subluxation of the radial head may be accomplished by supinating the forearm or extending the elbow while placing the thumbs over the radial head. (*3, p 1765*)

6.18 (C) Volkmann's ischemic contracture is a serious complication of supracondylar fracture from arterial ischemia. General signs of ischemia would be present. (*3, p 1766*)

6.19 (C) These findings are consistent with a rupture of the biceps, particularly the finding of an egg-shaped mass. (*3, p 1769*)

6.20 (E) The radial nerve supplies the muscles that extend the wrist. (*3, p 1770*)

6.21 (A) The distal radius is the bone most frequently fractured in wrist injuries. (*3, p 1774*)

6.22 (D) Scaphoid fractures are the most common carpal fractures. (*3, p 1778*)

6.23 (B) The patient with a displaced femoral neck fracture will not be able to bear weight and will have a shortened, externally rotated leg. (*3, p 1809*)

6.24 (B) The medial meniscus is about twice as likely to be torn as the lateral. (*3, p 1819*)

6.25 (D) Stable single-ligament injuries can best be treated conservatively with follow-up orthopedic referral. (*3, p 1819*)

6.26 (B) Cessation of the offending activity for a sufficient period of time is the recommended treatment for shin splints. (*3, p 1824*)

6.27 (C) Chemical cauterization after aspiration followed by a compression bandage is the suggested initial treatment of wrist ganglion cysts. Surgery is the next option if this treatment fails. (*2, p 347*)

6.28 (E) A positive Yergason test (supination against resistance) and point tenderness over the tip of the acromion suggest bicipital tendinitis. (*2, p 349*)

6.29 (B) Rupture of the Achilles tendon causes inability to toe walk, weak plantar flexion, and often a palpable gap along the course of the tendon. (*3, p 352*)

6.30 (E) Frozen shoulder, or adhesive capsulitis, commonly occurs in the elderly and limits passive ROM. (*2, p 350*)

6.31 (B) About 50% of patients with mechanical low back pain will be better in 2 wk. About 90% are better in 4 wk; thus few progress to chronic pain syndromes. (*2, p 367*)

6.32 (C) Multiple myelomas are the most common primary bone tumors. (*2, p 369*)

6.33 (C) Degenerative changes are present in many patients over 40 years of age and do not have good correlation with symptoms. (*2, p 370*)

6.34 (C) A pars defect is most common cause of low back pain in this age group. (*2, p 368*)

6.35 (C) The nodules described are Bouchard's nodes due to bony overgrowth associated with osteoarthritis. (*4, p 514*)

6.36 (D) Median nerve entrapment causes thenar atrophy. (*4, p 515*)

6.37 (C) Bacteria may be able to penetrate seemingly intact skin to attack the olecranon bursa. (*1, p 822*)

6.38 (A) The more powerful, fluorinated steroid preparations are best suited for deep injection to minimize risk of skin atrophy. (*1, p 831*)

6.39 (E) Amitriptyline in doses lower than those used to treat depression has proven helpful in treating fibromyalgia, probably by treating the underlying sleep disorders. (*1, p 820*)

6.40 (D) The medial collateral ligament often suffers from valgus stress secondary to a direct blow to the lateral knee, making it the most commonly injured ligament in the knee. (*3, p 1817*)

References

1. Tierney LM, McPhee SJ, Papadakis MA (eds): *Current Medical Diagnosis & Treatment,* 39/e, New York, McGraw-Hill, 2000.

2. Moser RL: *Primary Care for Physician Assistants,* New York, McGraw-Hill, 1998.

3. Tintinalli JF, Kelen GD, Stapczynski JS: *Emergency Medicine: A Comprehensive Study Guide,* 5/e, New York, McGraw-Hill, 2000.

4. Bickley LS, Hoekelman RA: *Bates' Guide to Physical Examination and History Taking,* 7/e, Philadelphia, Lippincott, 1999.

7

Rheumatology

Larry Dennis, PA-C, MPAS

DIRECTIONS (Questions 7.1–7.30): Each of the numbered items or incomplete statements in this chapter is followed by answers or completions of the statement. Select the **one** lettered answer or completion that is **best** in each case.

7.1 All the following laboratory and radiologic findings are consistent with the diagnosis of osteoarthritis **EXCEPT**
   A. Normal erythrocyte sedimentation rate
   B. Joint space narrowing, osteophytes, and subchondral sclerosis
   C. Elevated antinuclear antibody test
   D. Clear synovial fluid on joint aspiration

7.2 Widespread musculoskeletal pain, fatigue, normal laboratory studies, and tenderness to palpation in at least 11 of 18 specific sites are characteristic of
   A. Polymyalgia rheumatica
   B. Fibrositis (fibromyalgia)
   C. Rheumatoid arthritis
   D. Polymyositis

7.3 A finger deformity commonly seen in rheumatoid arthritis that presents with flexion of the proximal interphalangeal joint and hyperextension of the distal interphalangeal joint is
  A. Dupuytren's contracture
  B. Swan neck deformity
  C. Trigger finger
  D. Boutonniere deformity

7.4 All of the following medications are used in the treatment of rheumatoid arthritis **EXCEPT**
  A. Colchicine
  B. Gold salts
  C. Methotrexate
  D. Aspirin

7.5 Bilateral leg weakness or saddle area anesthesia, loss of bowel or bladder control, or impotence as chief complaints in a patient with a history of back pain should alert the clinician to the possibility of
  A. Cauda equina syndrome
  B. L_3 lumbar radiculopathy
  C. Peripheral neuropathy
  D. Meralgia paresthetica

7.6 A 17-year-old boy presents with complaints of a painful, swollen, atraumatic knee. The knee appears erythematous and feels warm to the touch. The green joint aspirate is reported back with a group III synovial fluid analysis. The physician assistant's next action should be
  A. Reassurance and rest
  B. Intraarticular steroid injection
  C. IV antibiotics
  D. Urgent referral to an orthopedist

7.7 A patient presenting with the acute onset of atraumatic, monoarticular ankle pain that is exquisite and prevents the patient from ambulating has a normal (<7.5 mg/dL) serum uric acid at the initial office visit. This lab result excludes the diagnosis of gouty arthritis.
  A. True
  B. False

7.8 In a patient presenting with an L₅ radiculopathy, the clinician might expect all of the following physical findings **EXCEPT**
   A. Weak great toe dorsiflexion
   B. Paresthesias in the medial forefoot
   C. Positive straight-leg raising test
   D. Loss of knee jerk tendon reflex

7.9 In assessing the sensory function in the fingers of a patient with carpal tunnel syndrome, the most sensitive clinical test to detect subtle differences between the affected and unaffected sides is
   A. Phalen test
   B. Tinel sign
   C. Two-point discrimination
   D. Carpal compression test

7.10 Edematous, proliferative synovium with an overlying layer of inflammatory exudate called a pannus is found in which arthritis?
   A. Systemic lupus erythematosus
   B. Rheumatoid arthritis
   C. Osteochondritis dissecans
   D. Scleroderma

7.11 The antinuclear antibody (ANA) lab test in systemic lupus erythematosus is _____ but not _____.
   A. Sensitive; specific
   B. Specific; sensitive
   C. Relative; essential

7.12 A disorder in which 90% of patients are women, in which dryness of the eyes and mouth occurs, and that may be associated with rheumatoid arthritis or other connective tissue diseases is
   A. Felty syndrome
   B. Sjögren syndrome
   C. Sequard syndrome
   D. Horner syndrome

7.13 The joint pattern of involvement has diagnostic value in the rheumatologic disorders and includes which of the following?
A. Inflammation
B. Number of joints involved
C. Type of joint involved
D. A and B
E. B and C

7.14 Pseudogout crystals appear _____ under compensated polariscopic examination, while the crystals of gout appear _____.
A. Negatively birefringent; birefringent
B. Birefringent; negatively birefringent

7.15 The findings of thinned skin with loss of joint skin creases, burning pain that seems exaggerated to the clinician, and pallor in the hand of a patient who had sustained minor trauma to the same hand 1 mo earlier would suggest the most likely diagnosis of
A. Peripheral neuropathy
B. Scleroderma
C. Reflex sympathetic dystrophy
D. Sudeck's atrophy

7.16 In rheumatoid arthritis, splinting is a nonpharmacologic therapy. Which of the following is a principle in splinting **NOT** to be utilized?
A. Splints are applied for the shortest time needed.
B. Fingers and hands should be in full extension at night.
C. Splints should be easily removable for range of motion.
D. Ankle splints should be at right angles.

7.17 In the drug category of NSAIDs, _____ may produce gastrointestinal ulceration, whereas selective _____ produce a lower incidence of endoscopic gastrointestinal ulceration.
A. COX-1 inhibitors; COX 2 inhibitors
B. COX-2 inhibitors; COX-1 inhibitors

7.18 Before making a final diagnosis of systemic lupus erythematosus, it is imperative to make sure the patient's condition has not been caused by
A. Actinic allergy
B. Syphilis
C. Lyme disease
D. A drug

7.19 An important cause of headache that classically presents with scalp tenderness, visual symptoms, and jaw claudication must be urgently investigated because it may lead to permanent blindness. This disease is
A. Amaurosis fugax
B. Temporal arteritis
C. Migraine
D. Tic douloureux

7.20 All of the following are considered to be seronegative spondyloarthropathies **EXCEPT**
A. Ankylosing spondylitis
B. Reiter syndrome
C. Colitic arthritis
D. Palindromic rheumatism

7.21 A patient presents with "sausage" appearance of the fingers and an arthritis that prominently affects the distal interphalangeal joints of the fingers. The patient complains of low back pain, but also has a negative rheumatoid factor. Which of the following is the most likely diagnosis?
A. Behçet syndrome
B. Psoriatic arthritis
C. Ankylosing spondylitis
D. HIV-associated arthritis

7.22 Also called "reactive arthritis," _____ typically presents clinically with urethritis, conjunctivitis, mucocutaneous lesions, and arthritis.
A. Lyme disease
B. Chlamydia arthritis
C. Reiter syndrome
D. Rheumatic fever

7.23 Which of the following disorders would **NOT** present with a manifestation of colitic arthritis?
A. Irritable bowel syndrome
B. Whipple's disease
C. Crohn's disease
D. Ulcerative colitis

7.24 Chondrocalcinosis on radiography is diagnostic of gouty arthritis.
A. True
B. False

7.25 What medical condition is most frequently produced in the lumbar spine by osteophytes of the facet joints, ligamentum flavum hypertrophy, and bulging or protrusion of the intervertebral disc?
A. Spondylolysis
B. Pott's disease
C. Still's disease
D. Spinal stenosis

7.26 A patient with a history of alcohol abuse presents with nodular, cordlike thickening of the palms, especially at the bases of the ring and small fingers. The most likely diagnosis would be
A. Stenosing tenosynovitis
B. Dupuytren's contracture
C. Polyfibrositis
D. Fibromyalgia

7.27 A patient may be classified as having systemic lupus erythematosus if the patient has at least 4 of 11 standard criteria. Which of the following is **NOT** one of the standard criteria?
A. Thrombocytosis
B. Photosensitivity
C. Serositis
D. Arthritis

7.28 A female patient presents with thickened skin with loss of normal folds, telangiectasias, and fingertip ulceration. Her chief complaint, however, is of difficulty swallowing. What is the most likely diagnosis?

A. Rheumatoid arthritis
B. Polymyalgia rheumatica
C. Systemic sclerosis
D. Wegener's granulomatosis

7.29 A teenage Boy Scout presents with headache accompanied by a stiff neck, arthralgias, myalgias, and an expanding, raised, red skin lesion that clears centrally as it expands. What disease must be prudently considered in the differential diagnosis?
A. Systemic lupus erythematosus
B. Leptospirosis
C. Lyme disease
D. Chagas disease

7.30 In gouty arthritis, colchicine may be used for the acute attack, but it may not be used to prevent future attacks.
A. True
B. False

Rheumatology

Answers and Discussion

7.1 (C) Osteoarthritis is a degenerative process and is not characterized as an autoimmune disease with positive serology. (*1, p 808*)

7.2 (B) Fibrositis is a common rheumatic disorder of unknown cause. There is an absence of objective findings and of diagnostic laboratory tests. (*1, p 820*)

7.3 (D) Boutonniere deformity is often confused with swan neck deformity, which presents with hyperextension of the proximal interphalangeal joint and flexion of the distal interphalangeal joint. (*1, p 827*)

7.4 (A) Colchicine is used in the treatment of gouty arthritis. (*1, pp 829–832*)

7.5 (A) Large or rapidly evolving neurologic deficits should also alert the clinician regarding cauda equina syndrome, which requires urgent evaluation for possible surgical intervention. (*1, p 819*)

7.6 (D) A group III synovial fluid analysis is purulent. Group I is noninflammatory, whereas group II is inflammatory History, exam, and laboratory data in this patient indicate a septic joint that requires immediate intervention by an orthopedist. (*1, p 808*)

7.7 **(B)** In up to 25% of cases a single uric acid determination is normal. Serial serum uric acid measurements reveal elevation in up to 95% of patients during an attack of gout. (*1, p 811*)

7.8 **(D)** Loss of knee jerk reflex might occur in L_4 radiculopathy. There is no commonly performed deep tendon reflex in the L_5 nerve root distribution. (*1, p 818*)

7.9 **(C)** The Phalen test, Tinel sign, and carpal compression test may all be performed in carpal tunnel syndrome, but the most sensitive clinical test is two-point discrimination. Electromyography and nerve conduction tests are special examinations that may be confirmatory. (*1, p 821*)

7.10 **(B)** Rheumatoid arthritis (RA) is a chronic, systemic inflammatory process that mainly affects the synovial membranes of joints. The etiology is unknown, but RA is classified as an autoimmune disease. (*1, pp 826–827*)

7.11 **(A)** The ANA is positive in nearly all patients with SLE, but it is also positive in many other conditions such as rheumatoid arthritis, diffuse scleroderma, polymyositis, and some forms of hepatitis. (*1, p 835*)

7.12 **(B)** Sjögren's syndrome is characterized by dry mouth and eyes (the sicca components). It is an autoimmune disease and is the result of chronic dysfunction of the exocrine glands. (*1, p 840*)

7.13 **(D)** Characteristics of the joint pattern in rheumatologic disorders include inflammation, number of joints involved, and site of joint involvement. (*1, p 807*)

7.14 **(B)** Rhomboid-shaped pseudogout crystals are blue when parallel to the polarized light and yellow when perpendicular, while the needle-shaped uric acid crystals of gout are the opposite. (*1, p 814*)

7.15 (C) RSD presents as a syndrome of vasomotor instability, trophic skin changes such as skin atrophy and hyperhidrosis, and pain and swelling in an extremity. (*1, p 822*)

7.16 (B) Hands and fingers should be night-splinted in the position of optimum function. Splints in RA provide relief from pain, help prevent contractures, and provide rest for the affected joints. (*1, p 829*)

7.17 (A) Cyclooxygenase (COX) is the enzyme that converts arachidonic acid to prostaglandins. COX-1 is important for the beneficial effects (including gastric protection) of prostaglandins, and COX-2 is important in the tissue inflammatory response. (*1, p 829*)

7.18 (D) Many pharmacologic agents (such as procainamide, hydralazine, and isoniazid) have been associated with a lupus-like syndrome. (*1, p 834*)

7.19 (B) Amaurosis fugax, "fleeting blindness," is characteristically caused by emboli, while temporal arteritis and migraine do not cause permanent blindness. Temporal arteritis is also known as giant cell arteritis. (*1, pp 843, 208*)

7.20 (D) Palindromic rheumatism is a disease of unknown origin, of usually normal lab values, and of recurring attacks of inflamed joints. Ankylosing spondylitis, Reiter syndrome, colitic arthritis, and psoriatic arthritis are the seronegative spondyloarthropathies. (*1, pp 846, 857*)

7.21 (B) Psoriatic arthritis and osteoarthritis are the only two diseases that cause prominent involvement of the DIP joints of the fingers. The "sausage" appearance of the fingers and toes and the negative rheumatoid factor suggest psoriatic arthritis. Also look for the typical psoriasis skin lesions and pitting of the fingernails. Sacroiliac joint involvement is common. (*1, pp 807, 848*)

7.22 (C) Reiter syndrome is of unknown etiology and is seronegative, although it is associated with HLA-B27 in 80% of white patients and 50% to 60% of black patients. Most cases occur days or weeks after a dysenteric infection or a sexually trans- mitted disease. This disease mimics several other arthritides, and a careful differential diagnosis is necessary. (*1, p 849*)

7.23 (A) Irritable bowel syndrome is of unknown etiology and does not present with arthritis. Whipple's disease, Crohn's disease, and ulcerative colitis are inflammatory bowel dis- eases and may present with arthritis. (*1, p 850*)

7.24 (B) Chondrocalcinosis is the deposition of calcium- containing salts in cartilage, not urate crystals as in gout. Chondrocalcinosis may be a radiographic feature of pseudo- gout. (*1, p 814*)

7.25 (D) Spinal stenosis may produce symptoms of low back pain or trouble with walking. Most patients with spinal stenosis are over age 60 years. The lower extremity symp- toms are known as pseudoclaudication and must be differen- tiated from true claudication. (*1, p 819*)

7.26 (B) Dupuytren's contracture is a disorder that is typified by nodular hyperplasia of the palmar fascia with contracture formation. The cause is unknown, but the condition is com- mon and occurs mainly in white men over the age of 50 years. (*1, p 821*)

7.27 (A) Thrombocytopenia is a criterion in the list of hemato- logic disorders, but thrombocytosis is not. Other criteria include malar rash, discoid rash, oral ulcers, renal disease, neurologic disease, immunologic abnormalities, and a posi- tive antinuclear antibody. (*1, p 834*)

7.28 (C) Systemic sclerosis is characterized by diffuse fibrosis of the internal organs and skin. The disease appears more fre- quently in women than men, and it usually appears in the third to fifth decades of life. Dysphagia is common. (*1, p 837*)

7.29 (C) Lyme disease is a tick-borne disease caused by the spirochete *Borrelia burgdorferi*. The skin lesion, erythema migrans, is typical of Lyme disease, but the clinical presen- tation of Lyme disease may be greatly varied. (*1, p 1391*)

7.30 (B) Colchicine may be used in acute attacks of gouty arthritis, but NSAIDs are generally preferred because the incidence of GI side effects with colchicine is so high. Colchicine may be used to prevent future attacks, and it may also be used to prevent an acute gouty attack when uricosurics or allopurinol are begun. (*1, p 813*)

Reference

1. Tierney LM, McPhee SJ, Papadakis MA (eds): *Current Medical Diagnosis & Treatment,* 39/e, New York, McGraw-Hill, 2000.

8

Obstetrics and Gynecology

Vickie S. Etzel, PA-C

Directions (Questions 8.1–8.60): Each of the numbered items or incomplete statements in this chapter is followed by answers or completions of the statement. Select the **one** lettered answer or completion that is **best** in each case.

Case: A 21-year-old Hispanic woman, G1 P0 Ab0 LC0, presents for her third prenatal visit. Her prenatal course has been uneventful and her labs are up to date and normal. She is 24 wk pregnant and reports sharp, stabbing pain in the lower abdominal area bilaterally when she quickly stands up or rolls over in bed. The pain lasts about 10 s. She denies vaginal bleeding or pressure in her lower abdomen. Fetal movement has been normal.

8.1 The most likely diagnosis is
   A. Braxton-Hicks contractions
   B. Round ligament pain
   C. Preterm labor
   D. Placenta abruptio

8.2 This condition warrants
  A. Reassurance and positional modification
  B. An ultrasound
  C. Observation in labor and delivery
  D. A β-hCG blood test

Case: A 31-year-old Caucasian woman, G2 P1 Ab (elective) 1 LC0, presents to your clinic. She reports her LMP was 8 wk ago, and it was shorter than usual. She has not had a pregnancy test, and has not been on birth control. She had an IUD a year ago. She is married and has been sexually active for the last year with her spouse only. She complains of spotting and mild to moderate pain in her lower abdomen for the last week. She has not had any signs of pregnancy. She had a history of PID in high school. Her vital signs are normal and she appears in no distress. You perform a pelvic exam and find that the Chadwick sign is absent, the uterus is anterior and normal in size, and there is a slightly tender and thickened area in the right adnexa. You collect specimens for a Pap and for chlamydia and GC screen.

8.3 The next test you should perform is
  A. KUB
  B. Urine hCG pregnancy test
  C. Culdocentesis
  D. Ultrasound

8.4 The test you performed in question 8.3 is positive. Your working diagnosis should be
  A. Kidney stone
  B. Ectopic pregnancy
  C. Menstrual cramps
  D. Ovarian mass

8.5 The next step calls for
  A. A urology consult
  B. Serum quantitative β-hCG, CBC, and consult with supervising physician
  C. Reassuring and sending the patient home on ibuprofen (600 mg q4h)
  D. Preparing the patient for an exploratory laparoscopy

8.6 Which of the following does **NOT** place a pregnant woman at risk for preterm labor?
   A. Cervicitis
   B. African American heritage
   C. O negative blood type
   D. Polyhydramnios

8.7 Which of the following is **NOT** a diagnostic criterion for preterm labor?
   A. Documented cervical change to 2 cm dilatation and 80% effacement
   B. 37-wk gestation
   C. Documented contractions at four per 20 min by external monitor
   D. 36-wk gestation

Case: A 23-year-old Asian woman, G1 P0 Ab0, presents to your ER and reports that she is 27 wk pregnant and that she had her first prenatal visit at the local health clinic 3 days ago. For the past 2 days, she has noted a dull pain in her lower back, which has since become constant. She also complains of fever the night before. The fever abated "some" with Tylenol, the last dose of which she took 6 h ago. She reports nausea and vomiting, and says she may have the flu. She denies vaginal bleeding, diarrhea, loss of vaginal fluid, dysuria, abdominal pain, or headache. She appears ill. Her vitals are: T = 102.5°F, P = 130 bpm, RR = 16 breaths/min. You also note right CVA tenderness and general discomfort over the lower abdomen. UA reveals 2+ leucocytosis and 1+ nitrites. At this point, you suspect acute pyelonephritis.

8.8 You should plan to
   A. Discharge the patient home on nitrofurantoin (100 mg bid for 10 days)
   B. Perform additional lab tests before you send her home on nitrofurantoin
   C. Admit her
   D. Do none of the above

8.9 Which of the following conditions places a woman at risk for pyelonephritis?

A. Polyhydramnios
B. Undiagnosed asymptomatic UTI
C. Early entry to prenatal care
D. Rh-negative blood type

8.10 Acute cholecystitis occurs in approximately 1:4000 pregnancies. Which of the following is **NOT** a risk factor for cholecystitis in a pregnant woman?
A. Vegetarian diet
B. Multigravidity
C. Pregnancy at age 39
D. Obesity
E. Prior use of estrogen-containing birth control pills

8.11 Which vaccine is considered safe to administer to a pregnant woman?
A. MMR
B. Oral polio
C. Tetanus
D. Smallpox

8.12 Combination oral contraceptives are indicated in conditions other than birth control. In which of the following are these agents **NOT** indicated?
A. Recurrent benign ovarian cysts
B. Endometriosis
C. Chronic anovulation
D. Suspected breast cancer

8.13 A progestin-only contraceptive (Norplant, Depo-Provera, progestin-only pill) is **MOST** appropriate for a
A. 25-year-old female with chronic active hepatitis C
B. 32-year-old female with IDDM and retinopathy
C. 28-year-old with history of DVT during her most recent pregnancy
D. 40-year-old female smoker (one ppd) who is 120 lb overweight and has (controlled) HTN
E. Any of the above

8.14 Which birth control method has the highest reported unplanned pregnancy rate with typical use?
   A. Male condoms only
   B. Diaphragm
   C. IUD
   D. Birth control pills

8.15 Which patient is at highest risk for cervical cancer?
   A. A 20-year-old virgin who is a nonsmoker
   B. A 22-year-old patient with a history of HPV and 2-year history of cigarette smoking
   C. A 24-year-old nonsmoker, sexually active at age 18 with one lifetime partner
   D. A 35-year-old nonsmoker with history of two partners lifetime, normal pap smears

8.16 A 34-wk-pregnant patient calls your office to report she was exposed to a child with varicella (chickenpox). She has neither had this illness in the past nor been vaccinated for it. She was exposed this morning. You
   A. Reassure her that she is 6 wk from delivery and, were she to develop chickenpox, it would run its course prior to delivery
   B. Reassure her that most adults have had this illness and that she can't be reinfected
   C. Recommend she have the varicella IgG titer ordered stat (test comes back in 24 h); if the test is negative, offer her varicella zoster immune globulin (VZIG)
   D. Consult with your physician
   E. Both C and D

8.17 Which of the following tests need **NOT** be ordered on a new OB low-risk prenatal patient with a negative PMH?
   A. Hepatitis B surface antigen
   B. RPR screen
   C. UA and C&S of urine
   D. Blood type and Rh and antibodies (DAT, IDC)
   E. Chem 20 panel

8.18 Which of the following would **NOT** be considered a risk factor for preterm labor?
   A. Yeast infection
   B. Twin gestation
   C. Third-trimester vaginal bleeding
   D. Known uterine anomaly

8.19 The corpus luteum produces this hormone that maintains pregnancy
   A. FSH
   B. Estrogen
   C. Progesterone
   D. LH

8.20 Which hormone stimulates uterine contractions?
   A. Oxytocin
   B. Prostaglandins
   C. Estradiol
   D. Both and B ιA
   E. Both B and C

8.21 Which hormone is used to determine whether or not a female is pregnant?
   A. Prostaglandins
   B. Estrogen
   C. Progesterone
   D. Human chorionic gonadotropin (hCG)

8.22 Two hormones that are used in many birth control pills, and that serve as a negative feedback loop to the hypothalamus, are
   A. Estradiol (estrogen)
   B. Human gonadotropin hormone
   C. Luteinizing hormone
   D. Progesterone
   E. Both B and C
   F. Both A and D

8.23 A 32-year-old woman presents at 26 wk of gestation for a prenatal visit. She tells you her first child weighed 9 lb and the second was born with spina bifida. Which one test would you order at this time?
A. Toxoplasmosis titer
B. CBC
C. 50-g glucose challenge
D. Triple screen (α-fetoprotein)

8.24 A 17-year-old woman presents to your clinic for a sports physical. She has a history of asthma and irregular periods. Her LMP, which was 60 days earlier, lasted only 2 days. You perform a pelvic exam and notice a bluish hue to her cervix. You suspect
A. Cardiac disease
B. Early pregnancy
C. Pulmonary disease
D. Cervical cancer

8.25 A 30-year-old Hispanic pregnant patient complains of a brown rash on her cheeks. You examine her and
A. Draw blood for ANA
B. Do an RPR screen
C. Refer her to a dermatologist
D. Recommend she avoid prolonged exposure to the sun

8.26 As you enter the exam room, the 14-year-old patient, who is 30 wk pregnant, tells you she is upset because she has waited too long to see you. You notice her BP is 132/90. Her baseline is 110/60. She has 1+ protein in her urine and her hands and feet are swollen. Your working diagnosis would be
A. Labile blood pressure due to stress
B. Chronic hypertension
C. Preeclampsia
D. Eclampsia

8.27 A 36-wk-pregnant patient complains of lack of fetal movement for the past day. On exam, FHR is 148 bpm. What test should you conduct?
A. Ultrasound
B. Oxytocin challenge

C. Nonstress test
D. None

8.28 A 28-year-old white woman presents to your ER complaining of lower abdominal pain that is aggravated by intercourse, especially after her most recent menses. She has had a temperature of 101.0°F the last 2 days, mild nausea without vomiting, and a cloudy vaginal discharge. She and her partner were treated for gonorrhea 6 mo ago. Your differential diagnosis should include
  A. Ectopic pregnancy
  B. Appendicitis
  C. Pelvic inflammatory disease
  D. Urinary tract infection
  E. All the above

8.29 Which test would **NOT** be indicated in this case?
  A. CBC
  B. Gonorrhea and chlamydia cultures
  C. Urine pregnancy test
  D. Strep throat screen
  E. Culdocentesis

8.30 Which of the following organisms is the most common cause of pelvic inflammatory disease?
  A. *Staphylococcus aureus*
  B. *Streptococcus viridans*
  C. *Neisseria gonorrhoeae*
  D. *Gardnerella vaginalis*
  E. Human papillomavirus

8.31 A 24-year-old Asian woman presents to your office for her yearly exam. She is concerned about growths on her vulva. She has a history of cervical dysplasia, which was treated with cryosurgery last year. Her last Pap smear was WNL. Which should you consider as the cause of the growth?
  A. *Herpes genitalis*
  B. *Chlamydia trachomatis*
  C. Hari Carter virus
  D. Human papillomavirus
  E. *G. vaginalis*

8.32 Which of the following medications can be used to treat *G. vaginalis* (bacterial vaginosis)?
   A. Ciprofloxacin
   B. Metronidazole
   C. Erythromycin
   D. Tetracycline
   E. Bicillin 2.4 million U

8.33 Which is **NOT** a risk factor for infertility?
   A. Male age 45
   B. Female history of pelvic inflammatory disease
   C. Low sperm count
   D. Female age 36

8.34 Which is **NOT** a sign of menopause?
   A. Vaginal mucus thinning
   B. Cessation of menses for greater than 1 year
   C. Atrophy of the uterus and cervix
   D. Hot flashes

8.35 Hormone replacement therapy protects against
   A. Osteoporosis
   B. Heart disease
   C. Skin and hair changes
   D. All of the above

8.36 A 24-year-old white woman presents to your office complaining of a progressive 2-year history of dyspareunia, pelvic pain, increased menstrual pain, and a history of infertility. Your differential diagnosis should include all of the following **EXCEPT**
   A. Endometriosis
   B. Urinary tract infection
   C. Pelvic adhesions
   D. Pelvic inflammatory disease

8.37 Causes of third-trimester vaginal bleeding include
   A. Placenta previa
   B. Uterine rupture
   C. Placenta abruptio
   D. Cervicitis
   E. All of the above

8.38 A 28-year-old black woman presents to your ER. She tells you she is pregnant and that she has not had time to see a doctor. She is 31 wk by LMP, and reports she has been spotting for 2 days. She also complains of a dull pain in her abdomen, and reports the baby has not been moving very well. Her vital signs are stable, and she is in no acute distress. The fetal heart rate is 152 bpm. Which test would be **LEAST** useful to assess this patient's complaint?
A. Urine pregnancy test
B. Vaginal speculum exam
C. Ultrasound of uterus
D. Bimanual exam

8.39 A low-risk OB patient presents for her 28-wk prenatal visit. She has AB negative blood type. Which is **NOT** indicated in this case?
A. Hematology consult
B. Antibody test
C. Rhogam IM injection
D. Counseling regarding prevention of hemolytic disease of the newborn

8.40 Which is the most common cause of infectious mastitis?
A. *Staphylococcus epidermidis*
B. *S. aureus*
C. *S. viridans*
D. *Streptococcus pyogenes*

8.41 A 34-year-old white woman presents to your office for a problem visit. She reports that while performing her monthly breast exam, she found a small nontender mass in the LUQ of her left breast. She reports she has a history of fibrocystic disease and that she smokes. You examine her and find a mobile nontender 1.0 × 1.0-cm mass in the LUQ of her left breast. What should you do next?
A. Reassure her it is probably fibrocystic breast disease.
B. Have her monitor it and return in 1 mo.
C. Order a mammogram.
D. None of the above

8.42 A 31-year-old Hispanic woman presents to your clinic complaining of a vaginal discharge that has been present for 1 wk. She is sexually active and reports having one partner for the past 2 years. The discharge is yellow and has an odor. She has used an OTC vaginal antifungal but the symptoms have not resolved. She is taking an oral contraceptive and states she is compliant. Her LMP was 2 wk ago. Which test should you perform with her exam?
  A. Gonorrhea test
  B. Chlamydia test
  C. Wet prep
  D. All of the above

8.43 You perform the test in question 8.42 and note clue cells and a positive KOH whiff test. What are your diagnosis and treatment?
  A. Monilia vaginitis; metronidazole 250 mg tid × 7 days
  B. Gardnerella vaginitis; metronidazole 250 mg tid × 7 days
  C. Gonorrhea; rocephin 250 mg IM
  D. Monilia vaginitis; fluconazole 75 mg once

8.44 The virus that causes dome-shaped umbilicated lesions is
  A. Herpes simplex I
  B. Condyloma acuminata
  C. Herpes zoster
  D. Molluscum contagiosum

8.45 A 33-year-old white woman presents to your office for her annual well woman exam. She complains she and her husband have been trying to have a baby for over 2 years. She reports having had irregular periods with amenorrhea spanning up to 6 mo throughout her life. Her LMP was 2 mo ago. She also reports that her periods are sometimes painful. She admits being "a little heavy" her whole life. You note hair growth on her upper lip, chin, side of face, chest, breasts, and abdomen. The hair is coarse and dark. The patient weighs 243 pounds and is 5'5" tall. You do not note any abnormalities on her pelvic exam even though it is limited due to her habitus. Which is the most likely working diagnosis?
  A. Secondary amenorrhea
  B. Infertility

C. Polycystic ovary syndrome (PCOS)
D. Thyroid dysfunction

8.46 In which of the following patients is genetic evaluation **NOT** indicated?
A. A 33-year-old female smoker
B. A 36-year-old primigravida
C. A 30-year-old woman who has a brother with muscular dystrophy
D. A 28-year-old woman with three spontaneous abortions fathered by the same man

8.47 During which trimester would you expect the maternal blood pressure to be the lowest?
A. First trimester
B. Second trimester
C. Third trimester
D. Blood pressure should be the same throughout pregnancy

8.48 A bluish or purplish color to the cervix is referred to as the
A. Hegar sign
B. Chadwick sign
C. Chloasma sign
D. Landin sign

8.49 You see a patient who is 24 wk pregnant. She complains of a red and pruritic papular rash on her abdomen for 1 wk. She says the rash worsens when she scratches her skin. She has had varicella, her rubella is negative, and she denies any contact with new substances. What is the most likely cause?
A. Measles
B. PUPPP
C. Scabies
D. Contact dermatitis

8.50 The maneuver used to determine fetal lie, presentation, and attitude is
A. Leopold maneuver
B. Brandt-Andrews maneuver
C. McRoberts maneuver
D. Ritgen maneuver

8.51 Which benign condition usually presents with abnormal uterine bleeding, infertility, spontaneous abortion, and, in some instances, lower uterine pressure and pain?
  A. Corpus luteum cyst
  B. Ectopic pregnancy
  C. Menopause
  D. Leiomyomas (fibroids)

8.52 A 60-year-old obese Caucasian woman presents to your office complaining of vaginal spotting. She is also a diabetic (type II) and hypertensive. She has been postmenopausal for 8 years. You suspect endometrial cancer. Which tests would help you in evaluation?
  A. Ultrasound of the uterus
  B. Endometrial biopsy
  C. Schiller test
  D. A and B
  E. B and C

8.53 Appropriate treatment of *Trichomonas vaginalis* calls for
  A. Douching
  B. Metronidazole for patient and partner
  C. Rocephin IM for patient and partner
  D. Bicillin IM for patient and partner

8.54 Which of the following can produce a vaginal discharge?
  A. Foreign bodies
  B. Chlamydia
  C. Candidiasis
  D. Trichomoniasis
  E. All of the above

8.55 Antibiotics considered appropriate in the treatment of chlamydia include
  A. Erythromycin-based
  B. Tetracycline
  C. Doxycycline
  D. Amoxicillin
  E. All of the above

8.56 Osteoporosis is loss of bone density without change in the bone's chemical composition. To manage osteoporosis in a healthy postmenopausal woman, you
  A. Prescribe conjugated estrogens (0.625 mg daily)
  B. Recommend calcium carbonate (1500 mg daily)
  C. Recommend a bone density scan
  D. A and B
  E. A, B, and C

8.57 You saw a 19-year-old female patient 3 days ago for a new visit. Her RPR titer is 1:64. You review her past visits and note her RPR was negative 8 mo ago. Her FTA-ABS (MHA-TP), now positive, was not indicated 8 mo ago. What is your diagnosis in this asymptomatic patient?
  A. Latent syphilis
  B. Primary syphilis
  C. Secondary syphilis
  D. Tertiary syphilis

8.58 How would you treat the patient in question 8.57 if she has no allergies?
  A. Benzathine penicillin G 2.4 million U by IM route
  B. Ampicillin 250 mg tid for 10 days
  C. Doxycycline 100 mg bid for 14 days
  D. Both A and B

8.59 Which of the following is **NOT** enhanced by smoking during pregnancy?
  A. Placenta abruptio
  B. Spontaneous abortion
  C. Low infant birth weight
  D. Large-for-gestational-age (LGA) babies

8.60 A woman presents to you for a pregnancy test. The test is positive. She tells you her LMP was April 26. You reach for your pregnancy wheel to give her a due date, but you cannot find it. Which rule do you use to give her a reliable EDC?
  A. Rule of 9s
  B. Glossmer's rule
  C. Nägele's rule
  D. Noland's rule

Obstetrics and Gynecology

Answers and Discussion

8.1 (B) Round ligament pain is a normal occurrence in pregnancy. Approximately 30% of pregnant women experience this late in the first trimester and throughout the second trimester. The pain is confined to the lower abdominal area over the ligament area. Sudden movement and changes in position produce the pain. Patients should be reassured that no tests are needed, and told that they should move slowly when changing position. (*1, p 178*)

8.2 (A) Reassurance and positional change suffice in cases of round ligament pain. (*1, p 178*)

8.3 (B) Urine hCG is usually positive within 10 days of conception. (*2, p 26*)

8.4 (B) The symptoms of ectopic pregnancy are sometimes vague. The Chadwick sign may be absent and the exam vague. The pain may be mildly to moderately severe. Bleeding can be irregular. Having had a diaphragm puts women at risk for infection and tubal scarring, as does a history of PID. (*1, p 732; 3, p 310*)

8.5 (B) The serum quantitative results must be correlated with suspected weeks of gestation, and the CBC needs to be performed to evaluate the patient's H/H due to the possibility of rupture. Consultation is critical as other tests need to be ordered and the patient may need observation for 23 h. This condition can sometimes be managed on an outpatient basis, but it can become emergent. Management depends on lab values and hemodynamic stability plus other factors. (*1, pp 732–735*)

8.6 (C) Blood type is not a risk factor for preterm labor. The other factors correlate with increased risk of uterine contractions prior to week 36. (*1, pp 750–752*)

8.7 (B) Labor is not considered preterm if it is prior to 20 wk or after 36 6/7 wk. (*2, p 808; 1, pp 759–760*)

8.8 (C) The patient should be admitted and managed as an inpatient. Her symptoms meet the criteria for pyelonephritis, which is treated with IV antibiotics for 48 h. She will need additional bloodwork and external fetal monitoring. Patients with this condition can become very ill and develop adult RDS, preterm labor, and systemic infection. Do not send these patients home. (*2, pp 1128–1130*)

8.9 (B) Undiagnosed asymptomatic UTI is a major reason for development of pyelonephritis. UA and C&S are used to identify pathogens that need coverage. Both are performed during the first prenatal visit. Blood type and amniotic fluid status are not risk factors for pyelonephritis. (*2, pp 1126–1127*)

8.10 (A) Vegetarian diet lowers the risk of acute cholecystitis somewhat because of lower fat and reduced bile production. The remaining answers are all risks for development of acute cholecystitis. (*1, pp 631–632*)

8.11 (C) Whereas tetanus toxoid is approved, the other agents listed are contraindicated during pregnancy. Smallpox is reportedly eradicated. (*4, pp 49, 522*)

8.12 (D) Suspected breast cancer is a contraindication to estrogen-containing medication. (*3, pp 411–412, 434*)

8.13 (E) Each of these conditions is a contraindication to estrogen pills. (*3, p 434*)

8.14 (B) Typical use shows a much higher rate of unplanned pregnancy than perfect use. Diaphragm, 20%; male condom only, 14%; pills, 5%; IUD, 0.1% to 2.0%. (*3, p 216*)

8.15 (B) Smoking and HPV increase the risk of cervical cancer greatly. The other patients are in a low- to no-risk category. (*3, p 51*)

8.16 (E) Varicella can cause pneumonia and other serious complications in the adult. (*4, p 579*)

8.17 (E) Chem panel is not indicated in a low-risk OB profile. (*5, p 75*)

8.18 (A) Yeast infection is not considered a risk factor for preterm labor. (*5, p 89*)

8.19 (D) The corpus luteum is maintained by hCG feedback. The corpus luteum produces estradiol and progesterone until the placenta is developed enough to produce steroids. Progesterone serves to maintain the pregnancy. Peak production occurs around 10 wk of gestation. (*1, p 44*)

8.20 (D) Both oxytocin and prostaglandins stimulate uterine contractions. (*1, p 121*)

8.21 (D) The developing trophoblast (to-be fetus) produces hCG. hCG is identical to LH and prevents menses by maintaining the corpus luteum cyst until 10 wk gestation. Most office tests will be positive 7 to 10 days after conception. (*1, pp 53–54*)

8.22 (F) Estradiol and progesterone are the hormones that perform this function. (*3, pp 405–106*)

8.23 (C) Large-for-gestational-age babies are born to mothers with uncontrolled diabetes. Stillbirth can also occur. An ultrasound may help assess spina bifida at this point. Triple screens are recommended from 15 to 20 wk gestation, but the best time is 16 to 18 wk. Toxoplasmosis titers are drawn if the patient has been exposed to cat litter. A CBC will not assess diabetes or spina bifida. (*2, pp 227–247*)

8.24 (B) The bluish hue is known as the Chadwick sign. To confirm your suspicion, you should perform a pregnancy test. (*6, p 186*)

8.25 (D) Chloasma is a normal hormonal change due to progesterone. The sun will deepen the pigment and make it more pronounced. It usually resolves postpartum. (*6, p 186*)

8.26 (C) The main signs and symptoms of preeclampsia are elevation of blood pressure to 160/110 or 30/15 from baseline, proteinuria, visual changes, headache, elevation in liver enzymes, thrombocytopenia (platelets < 100,000), and change in clotting studies. If not diagnosed and treated, this condition can lead to eclampsia (convulsions and DIC), which can be life-threatening. (*6, pp 380–395*)

8.27 (C) The nonstress test is the main test performed for fetal surveillance. It is reliable in the assessment of fetal outcome up to 5 days posttest. (*6, p 288*)

8.28 (E) These symptoms are vague and confusing. Ectopic pregnancy can be life-threatening. Any non-post-menopausal woman complaining of lower abdominal pain should have a pregnancy test performed to rule out pregnancy. Some of these conditions can occur simultaneously. (*6, pp 769–770*)

8.29 (D) Strep throat screen is not indicated. The other tests will help you rule in the diagnosis. (*6, p 770*)

8.30 (C) *N. gonorrheae* is the most common cause. (*6, p 770*)

8.31 (D)   Human papillomavirus causes wartlike growths and cervical dysplasia. The patient needs Pap smears at least yearly. (*6, p 696*)

8.32 (B)   Metronidazole (Flagyl) 500 mg twice daily for 5 to 7 days is the treatment of choice. (*6, p 697*)

8.33 (A)   Being a male over 45 years of age does not in itself add to infertility. (*6, pp 996–999*)

8.34 (D)   Hot flashes are a symptom, not a sign. (*6, pp 1033–1035*)

8.35 (D)   Hormone replacement therapy is indicated for protection against all the items listed. (*6, pp 1036–1049*)

8.36 (B)   The patient's condition may be due to each of the diseases listed. UTIs generally have a more acute course. (*6, pp 804–805*)

8.37 (E)   Each of the conditions listed can result in vaginal bleeding. (*6, p 399*)

8.38 (C)   You must rule out placenta previa before vaginal exams because a digital exam can lead to placenta disruption (if the placenta is covering the cervical os) and hemorrhage. (*6, p 339*)

8.39 (A)   Consulting a hematologist is not indicated. The patient is low risk. (*7, p 744*)

8.40 (B)   Of the agents listed, *S. aureus* is the most common cause of mastitis. (*7, pp 588–589*)

8.41 (C)   In view of the patient's risk factors, a mammogram is in order to rule out malignancies. (*7, pp 1124–1125*)

8.42 (C)   Wet prep is the main test to evaluate this discharge. If in doubt about monogamy, you could perform a GC/chlamydia test. (*6, p 691*)

8.43 (F)   Gardnerella vaginosis is a common vaginal infection. The fishy odor and clue cells are diagnostic of this infection.

It usually resolves with one course of treatment. Partners do not have to be treated unless recurrent infections are noted. (*6, pp 691, 699*)

8.44 (D) This description is characteristic of molluscum contagiosum. Treatment can include freezing, curettage, and chemical cauterization. (*6, p 705*)

8.45 (C) Polycystic ovary syndrome is the most likely cause. Amenorrhea and infertility are symptoms of this condition, which has been ongoing throughout this patient's life. Even though thyroid disease is less likely, testing for thyroid disease may be prudent, if it has not been done recently. (*8, p 679*)

8.46 (A) Smoking has nothing to do with genetic disorders. Any patient with a history of multiple miscarriages, especially fathered by the same man, may have an undiagnosed genetic condition. Women who will be 35 at delivery are at risk for genetic conditions. A patient with a family history of a first-degree relative with any genetic disorder should be offered genetic counseling and evaluation. (*8, pp 215, 220–221, 237*)

8.47 (B) There is a reduction of vascular resistance through the first 24 wk. This is most obvious during the second trimester (13 to 27 wk). (*8, pp 98–99; 6, p 150*)

8.48 (B) The color change of the cervix is due to increased blood flow during pregnancy. (*6, p 186*)

8.49 (B) Pruritic urticarial papules and plaques of pregnancy (PUPPP) is common and self-limiting. It usually begins on the abdomen. Treatment includes antihistamines and antipruritic medications. The condition has no ill effects on the fetus. (*6, p 476*)

8.50 (A) There are four distinct maneuvers to determine what is at the fundus, where the spine and small parts are, what is presenting in the pelvis, and where the cephalic prominence is. This is a part of the third-trimester prenatal visit. (*1, pp 377–378*)

8.51 (D)   Leiomyomas or fibroids are the most common complaints. On exam, one may note smooth spherical masses and distorted uterine contour. The uterus may be enlarged because of these lesions. (*6, pp 731–739*)

8.52 (D)   Ultrasound and endometrial biopsy are very helpful. The Schiller test is used in the evaluation of cervical dysplasia. The incidence is highest in the sixth and seventh decades. Obese, nulliparous, hypertensive, and diabetic patients are at higher risk. Estrogen is a contributing factor. (*6, p 937*)

8.53 (E)   Vaginal discharge may have various etiologies. A detailed history and a good exam plus thorough testing will help determine the cause. (*6, p 690*)

8.54 (B)   The only approved treatment is metronidazole, which can be used in pregnant women. The dose may vary from 250 mg tid for 7 days to 2 g taken all at once. Both patient and partner should be treated at the same time to prevent reinfection. (*6, p 699*)

8.55 (E)   Dosing varies with the product. In nonpregnant females, first-line therapy is tetracycline or doxycycline. In pregnant women, first-line therapy is erythromycin-based products. Ampicillin is used for those who cannot tolerate erythromycin. (*6, p 751*)

8.56 (D)   The therapy would be calcium carbonate and estrogen replacement. Bone density scans are used to assess the bone, but are not therapeutic. One woman in two is at risk for bone fracture in the postmenopausal years. Prevention is important, as bone mass loss begins as early as 30 to 35 years of age. (*6, pp 1036–1038; 1, pp 645–646*)

8.57 (A)   Latent syphilis occurs after the secondary stage symptoms resolve and may be life-long. Primary syphilis occurs 2 wk to 3 mo after exposure. A chancre or ulcer will appear Secondary syphilis occurs 2 wk to 6 mo after the chancre and can include rash and condylomalata. Tertiary syphilis is marked by destructive lesions of the skin and bone, cardiovascular system, or nervous system. It is fatal in 25% of those affected. (*8, pp 590–593*)

8.58 (D)   Benzathine, penicillin, and doxycycline are adequate treatments for primary, secondary, and latent (<1 year) syphilis. (*8, pp 590–594*)

8.59 (D)   Smoking should be discontinued during pregnancy in view of the risks listed. (*2, p 959*)

8.60 (C)   Nägele's rule is very reliable, at times more so than the calendars, which can be up to 5 days off. To determine the EDC by Nägele's Rule in this case, add 7 days to the LMP and then count back 3 mo. An LMP of April 26 would give an EDC of January 3. Normal pregnancies are 282 days on average. (*2, pp 229–230*)

References

1. Gabbe SG, Niebyl JR, Simpson JL (eds): *Obstetrics— Normal and Problem Pregnancies*, 3/e, London, Churchill Livingstone, 1996.

2. Cunningham FG, MacDonald PC, Gant NF, et al (eds): *Williams Obstetrics*, 20/e, Stamford, CT, Appleton & Lange, 1997.

3. Hatcher RA, Trussel J, Stewart F, et al: *Contraceptive Technology*, 17/e, revised, New York, Ardent Media, 1998.

4. American Academy of Pediatrics: *1997 Red Book: Report of the Committee on Infectious Diseases*, 24/e, 1997.

5. American Academy of Pediatrics: *Guidelines for Prenatal Care*, 4/e, 1997.

6. DeCherney AH, Pernoll ML: *Current Obstetrics and Gynecologic Diagnosis and Treatment*, 8/e, Norwalk, CT, Appleton & Lange, 1994.

7. Tierney LM Jr., McPhee SJ, Papadakis MA (eds): *Current Medical Diagnosis & Treatment*, 37/e, Stamford, CT, Appleton & Lange, 1998.

8. Benson RC, Pernoll M: *Handbook of Obstetrics and Gynecology*, 9/e, McGraw-Hill, 1994.

9

Cardiology

Karen S. Stephenson, MS, PA-C

DIRECTIONS (Questions 9.1–9.43): Each of the numbered items or incomplete statements in this chapter is followed by answers or completions of the statement. Select the **one** lettered answer or completion that is **best** in each case.

9.1 A 45-year-old man presents for a physical for life insurance at work. While there, his blood pressure (BP) is measured as 145/95; he is 20% over his ideal body weight. What would not be part of your initial response to his BP reading?
  A. Check previous BP measurements
  B. Check cuff size for appropriate diameter
  C. Start a beta blocker because the patient seems anxious
  D. Wait 2 to 5 min and repeat the measurement

9.2 When the patient returns 1 wk later, his blood pressure is recorded three times and the results average 147/98. His BP on previous visits over the last 5 years averaged 130/88, though his weight has gradually increased over that time. How would you begin the management of his elevated BP?
  A. Begin BP medication
  B. Determine stage of hypertension
  C. Evaluate for end organ damage
  D. Inquire about medical conditions

9.3 Which of the following medical conditions place this patient at highest risk for complications from his hypertension?
A. Angina
B. Diabetes
C. Hyperthyroidism
D. Obesity

9.4 Which of the following should be considered as initial evaluation for possible end organ damage?
A. BUN and creatinine
B. Echocardiogram
C. Electrocardiogram
D. Urinalysis

9.5 Because the patient is overweight, which of the following random plasma glucose levels should be considered an indication for further testing?
A. 140 mg/dL
B. 160 mg/dL
C. 180 mg/dL
D. 200 mg/dL

9.6 The patient's 2-h post load glucose level is 140 mg/dL, which is normal. Now that you have determined that your patient does not have diabetes, which of the following would be **MOST** appropriate?
A. Aerobic exercise
B. Dietary referral
C. Weight loss
D. All of the above

9.7 If the above described regimen does not bring your patient's blood pressure down to normal levels, which of the following would be an appropriate first drug choice?
A. ACE inhibitors
B. Beta blockers
C. Calcium antagonists
D. Diuretics

9.8 All of the following groups of persons with hypertension benefit from diuretics **EXCEPT**

A. African Americans
B. Type II diabetics
C. Diabetics with proteinuria
D. Elderly persons

9.9 A 65-year-old Hispanic woman is brought to your emergency room via ambulance at about 8:30 A.M. after a 2-h episode of diaphoresis and shortness of breath (SOB). She is a longtime patient of yours who took her medication for hypertension only occasionally because of the brisk diuresis and dizziness that occurred after taking the medication. She has refused to consider a change in her medication because she was "tired of taking medicines." Otherwise her health has been good until recently with her diagnosis of hypertension. Her only other medication includes NSAIDs for arthritis in both her knees from long years as a migrant farm worker. When she arrives, she appears in respiratory distress and is diaphoretic. She denies chest pain, arm pain, or jaw pain. She feels a little nauseated but is most concerned about the shortness of breath. There is no history of similar episodes. What medication should be given, considering the two most likely causes of her distress?
A. ACE inhibitors
B. Beta blockers
C. Calcium channel blockers
D. Diuretics

9.10 Which of the following treatments would not be included in the initial treatment of this patient?
A. Aspirin
B. Calcium channel blockers
C. Nitroglycerine
D. Oxygen by nasal prong

9.11 All of the following findings on the patient's ECG would indicate acute myocardial ischemia **EXCEPT**
A. Elevated ST segment
B. Inverted T wave
C. Inverted P wave
D. Q wave

9.12 Which of the following lab tests would **NOT** be helpful in identifying the cause(s) of the patient's SOB?
A. CPK-MB
B. LDH$_1$
C. SGOT
D. Troponins

9.13 Which of the above mentioned enzymes is **MOST** sensitive to cardiac damage?
A. CPK MB
B. LDH$_1$
C. SGOT
D. Troponins

9.14 You look at the patient's chest x-ray to determine if she has congestive heart failure (CHF). Which of the following is **NOT** consistent with CHF?
A. Cardiomegaly
B. Pleural effusions
C. Pulmonary venous congestion
D. Right middle lobe infiltrate

9.15 Which physical finding(s) would **NOT** support the diagnosis of CHF?
A. Jugular venous congestion
B. Periorbital edema
C. S$_3$ gallop
D. Tachycardia

9.16 Left-sided heart failure can also be divided into systolic and diastolic dysfunction. All but which of the following can be described as part of systolic dysfunction?
A. Low ejection fraction
B. Post-MI status
C. Q waves on ECG
D. S$_4$ gallop

9.17 Which of the following medications would be **MOST** appropriate for this elderly person with ST segment elevation on ECG, elevated cardiac troponins and congestive heart failure on exam and chest x-ray, and systolic dysfunction?

A. ACE inhibitor, diuretic, nitrates, and digitalis
B. ACE inhibitor, diuretic, nitrates, and verapamil
C. ACE inhibitor, diuretic, nitrates, and ionotropic agents

9.18 You start the patient on an ACE inhibitor. Which of the following side effects would you **NOT** expect from this medication?
A. Angioedema
B. Cough
C. Leucocytosis
D. Rash

9.19 You also decide to start the patient on digitalis for treatment of the CHF that developed with her myocardial infarction. Which of the following statements about digitalis is **NOT** true?
A. Digitalis is recommended for patients with CHF in normal sinus rhythm.
B. Digitalis should be given to those with an ejection fraction <30%.
C. Digitalis does not reduce mortality but reduces the number of hospital stays.
D. Low potassium and magnesium levels can lead to digitalis toxicity.

9.20 Which of the following drugs can be routinely administered to this patient who has just suffered a myocardial infarction?
A. Antiarrhythmic drugs
B. Aspirin
C. Calcium agonists
D. IV magnesium

9.21 You see your patient 2 days after her MI and auscultate a new murmur at the apex that occurs during systole and radiates to the axilla. What is this?
A. Aortic stenosis
B. Mitral stenosis
C. Mitral regurgitation
D. Tricuspid regurgitation

9.22 If you had heard a pericardial rub instead of the new murmur, what condition would you expect to have caused the rub?
   A. Aneurysm
   B. Embolism
   C. Pericarditis
   D. Ventricular septal defect

9.23 All of the following physical findings would lead you to consider that your patient is also suffering from cardiac tamponade **EXCEPT**
   A. Distended neck veins
   B. Elevated blood pressure
   C. Paradoxical pulses
   D. Tachycardia

9.24 A 60-year-old man presents to your clinic with a 2 × 2-cm ulcerated lesion on the medial aspect of his left ankle. He says it has been there for about 1 mo; he has been treating it with neomycin ointment without success. He reports a 42-pack-year history of tobacco use, and states that both his parents died from heart disease. He has not had a medical exam in 20 years and takes no OTC medications. What other signs would you **NOT** expect to find on exam?
   A. Cool extremity
   B. Edema
   C. Hyperpigmentation
   D. Venous varicosities

9.25 If the problem were arterial insufficiency, all of the following findings would be present **EXCEPT**
   A. Absent pulses
   B. Hair loss
   C. Pallor
   D. Warmth

9.26 The patient has told you he has also noticed some pain in his calf when walking; the pain is relieved with rest. What would be your preliminary diagnosis?
   A. Gangrene
   B. Intermittent claudication

C. Vasculitis
D. Venous varicosities

9.27 Which of the following is an invasive test needed to identify the location of the narrowed vessel?
A. Digital pulse volume reading
B. Doppler flow studies
C. Ultrasound
D. Venous catheterization

9.28 What is the most common cause of death in patients with peripheral vascular disease?
A. Asthma
B. Infection
C. Myocardial infarction
D. Stroke

9.29 Supportive measures for peripheral arterial disease include all of the following **EXCEPT**
A. Cigarette smoking
B. Daily foot care
C. Exercise
D. Lipid reduction

9.30 If you hear a holosystolic murmur of tricuspid regurgitation and notice stigmata of chronic lung disease such as barrel chest, wheezing throughout the lung fields, and cyanosis in this patient, what other condition must you suspect?
A. Congenital heart disease
B. Cor pulmonale
C. Rheumatic fever
D. Ventricular tachycardia

9.31 At what intercostal space would you expect to hear tricuspid regurgitation?
A. 2nd right
B. 2nd left
C. 4th left
D. 5th left

9.32 The hypoxia produced by COPD may also lead to all of the following **EXCEPT**
  A. Arrhythmias
  B. Jugular venous distension
  C. Right heart failure
  D. Reduced liver size

9.33 What cardiac arrhythmia would be closely related to the patient's generalized atherosclerosis, right heart failure, and chronic hypoxia?
  A. Atrial fibrillation
  B. Atrial flutter
  C. Premature ventricular beats
  D. First-degree heart block

9.34 When looking at the ECG to evaluate your patient in atrial fibrillation, what finding would indicate this arrhythmia?
  A. Absent P waves
  B. Bradycardia
  C. PVCs
  D. Tachycardia

9.35 Which of the following statements does **NOT** describe the management of atrial fibrillation?
  A. Begin an antiarrhythmic medication, quinidine-like drug.
  B. Consider cardioversion if the medication does not slow the pulse.
  C. Identify precipitating factors, such as thyrotoxicosis.
  D. Ignore the ventricular pulse.

9.36 Which of the following describes the manner in which the ventricular rate is slowed by digitalis?
  A. Prolonged refractory period of AV node
  B. Prolonged refractory period of SA node
  C. Shortened refractory period of AV node
  D. Shortened refractory period of SA node

9.37 Which of the following statements describes the murmur of aortic stenosis?
  A. Holosystolic murmur radiating to the axilla
  B. Diastolic murmur heard at the apical impulse

C. Systolic ejection murmur radiating to the carotids
D. Systolic ejection murmur heard at the left sternal border

9.38 Mitral stenosis produces which of the following murmurs?
A. Holosystolic murmur radiating to the axilla
B. Diastolic murmur heard at the apical impulse
C. Systolic ejection murmur radiating to the carotids
D. Systolic ejection murmur heard at the left sternal border

9.39 Both of these murmurs require evaluation. Which one of the following is not necessary for evaluation of the murmurs?
A. Cardiac catheterization
B. Complete blood count
C. Echocardiogram
D. Electrocardiogram

9.40 Which heart murmur is likely to be associated with an opening snap?
A. Aortic stenosis
B. Mitral stenosis
C. Pulmonary regurgitation
D. Tricuspid regurgitation

9.41 Mitral valve prolapse would produce a click in which part of the cardiac cycle?
A. Just prior to the first heart sound
B. Midsystole
C. Split of the second heart sound
D. Middiastole

9.42 Which of the following statements about mitral valve prolapse (MVP) is **NOT** true?
A. MVP tends to occur with other heart conditions such as rheumatic heart disease.
B. MVP stresses the papillary muscle, which then worsens the function of the mitral valve.
C. Severe cases may lead to mitral stenosis.
D. Ventricular arrhythmias may accompany the MVP, especially in serious cases.

9.43 Because there is such a wide range of symptoms, which of the following is not part of the care of a patient with MVP?

    A. Antibiotics to prevent infective endocarditis

    B. ACE inhibitors for chest pain

    C. Antiarrhythmics for ventricular arrhythmias

    D. Echocardiography to evaluate MVP

Cardiology

Answers and Discussion

9.1 (C) A diagnosis of hypertension should be based on several measurements over two or more visits, with the blood pressure taken several times and then averaged. (*1, p 2417*)

9.2 (B) Begin by ascertaining the stage of hypertension; per JNCVI recommendations, the patient would have stage 1 hypertension. (*1, p 2417*)

9.3 (B) Diabetes alone places the patient in risk group C with or without target organ damage such as angina. (*1, p 2420*)

9.4 (B) An echocardiogram would not be considered an initial evaluation. The patient also needs a chest x-ray, electrolytes, and an evaluation for diabetes. (*1, p 2419*)

9.5 (B) According to the 2000 recommendations, a random glucose of 160 mg/dL is high enough to indicate further testing for diabetes. The patient has three risk factors for diabetes: obesity > 20% body weight, age > 45 years, and hypertension > 140/90. He should be given the standard 75-g glucose load prior to testing. (*2*)

9.6 (D) Weight loss is an effective initial treatment for uncomplicated stage 1 hypertension. Aerobic exercise is an integral part of an effective weight loss program. Dietary changes include a low-fat diet with restricted protein and sodium as well as increased amounts of potassium. (*1, p 2422*)

9.7 (D) Diuretics, beginning at low doses, remain a good choice in treating hypertension because they reduce plasma volume and produce peripheral vasodilatation. It is important to prescribe the medication at a low dose and if possible as a long-acting once-daily dose initially so as to lower blood pressure gradually. (*1, p 2428*)

9.8 (C) African Americans and the elderly respond well to diuretics that potentiate other antihypertensive drugs. Diuretics are inappropriate for those with diabetes who have developed proteinuria. This group of diabetics should receive ACE inhibitors. (*1, pp 2429, 2433, 2435*)

9.9 (A) ACE inhibitors can serve to treat both acute MI and CHF. Adding beta blockers can further reduce the rate of mortality. (*3, p 38*)

9.10 (B) Calcium channel blockers have not been shown to decrease mortality post-MI and may even cause harm. (*4, pp 217, 221*)

9.11 (C) Elevated ST segments indicate the area of injury, inverted T waves indicate the area of ischemia, and Q waves indicate the area of infarction. (*4, p 214*)

9.12 (C) SGOT has been previously used to follow cardiac muscle injury and infarction. (*4, pp 216–217*)

9.13 (D) The two cardiac troponins—T and I—are specific for cardiac muscle damage. Troponin I can be used to identify non–Q wave myocardial infarctions; the higher the troponin level, the greater the damage to cardiac tissue. (*4, pp 216–217*)

9.14 (D) Right middle lobe infiltrates indicate pneumonia rather than congestive heart failure. (*4, p 241*)

9.15 (B) The other three findings are common ones for congestive heart failure. Other physical findings include tachypnea, rales, peripheral edema, hepatomegaly, and ascites. (*4, p 241*)

9.16 (D) An S_4 gallop is more common in diastolic dysfunction, which is likely to be associated with hypertension, valvular heart disease, or restrictive heart disease. The ECG in diastolic dysfunction shows LVH without a displaced PMI at exam or cardiomegaly on CXR. Both types of dysfunction demonstrate pulmonary congestion. Every person with congestive heart failure should have an echocardiogram to distinguish these two types of CHF. (*4, pp 237–238*)

9.17 (A) ACE inhibitors are useful for both CHF and AMI, as are diuretics and nitrates. Verapamil, as well as other calcium channel blockers, and positive ionotropic agents are not indicated in the treatment of either condition. It is vitally important that the CHF be classified as diastolic or systolic dysfunction. Medications such as ACE inhibitors, digitalis, and diuretics are contraindicated in some types of diastolic dysfunction, such as aortic stenosis, and IHSS. (*4, pp 241–242*)

9.18 (C) ACE inhibitors produce cough, angioedema, and rash, but not leucocytosis. (*4, p 242*)

9.19 (A) Digitalis is generally reserved for those in severe CHF, such as those with low ejection fractions. Quinidine and verapamil can also potentiate toxicity. Digitalis is compatible with diuretics and ACE inhibitors. (*4, p 242*)

9.20 (B) Magnesium should be given based on the person's magnesium level rather than routinely. Adequate magnesium levels are cardioprotective; they cause vasodilation, decrease platelet aggregation, and stabilize cell membranes. Calcium agonists, especially short-acting ones, may actually cause harm, and antiarrhythmic drugs are not routinely recommended. (*4, pp 220–221*)

9.21 (C) Mitral regurgitation appears during an acute MI secondary to papillary muscle dysfunction and indicates a worsening in the patient's condition that may require more intensive support to maintain blood pressure and lower pulmonary wedge pressure. (*4, pp 220–221*)

9.22 (C) Pericarditis is the most likely cause of the friction rub. The others are other complications following acute MI. (*4, p 252*)

9.23 (B) The blood pressure is low secondary to the impaired ability of the heart to pump blood. (*4, p 252*)

9.24 (A) Generally, the leg is warm to the touch in these cases because there is adequate arterial blood, but the incompetent venous valves lead to the edema in venous insufficiency. (*6, p 1405*)

9.25 (D) In arterial insufficiency, the extremity is usually cool because of the diminished arterial blood flow. Other findings include thickened nails, smooth and shiny skin, and muscle atrophy. (*6, p 1398*)

9.26 (B) Patients may also notice cramping, numbness, or a sense of fatigue. (*6, p 1398*)

9.27 (D) The others locate the occlusion by noninvasive techniques. (*6, p 1398*)

9.28 (C) Persons with peripheral vascular disease have atherosclerosis throughout their arterial tree and may also experience sudden death. (*6, p 1399*)

9.29 (A) The most important behavioral change for the person with peripheral arterial disease is smoking cessation. Smoking causes peripheral vasoconstriction, whereas exercise, especially walking, leads to vasodilatation and development of collateral circulation. Patients must pace themselves as they exercise to extend the distance they walk before pain occurs. (*6, p 1399*)

9.30 (B) COPD is the most common cause of cor pulmonale and is produced by pathologic changes in the lung's vasculature brought on by hypoxia, acidemia, and hypercarbia. (*7, pp 1326–1327*)

9.31 (C) The murmur of tricuspid regurgitation would be located at the 4th left intercostal space. (*8, p 330*)

9.32 (D) Generally the liver is enlarged as a part of right heart failure. The signs of right heart failure are difficult to separate from those of airway obstruction in the lung. (*7, p 1327*)

9.33 (A) Atrial fibrillation is brought on by hypoxia, hypercapnia, or acute insult. (*9, p 1264*)

9.34 (A) In atrial fibrillation, the atrium is unable to produce coordinated activity and thus the P wave is absent. (*9, p 1264*)

9.35 (D) In managing atrial fibrillation, the ventricular pulse must be reduced just as the atrial one must be. Digitalis, calcium channel blockers, and beta blockers can slow the rate. (*9, p 1265*)

9.36 (A) Digitalis prolongs the refraction in the AV node and slows conduction through it. (*9, p 1264*)

9.37 (C) This describes the murmur of aortic stenosis. (*10, p 1319*)

9.38 (B) This describes the murmur of mitral stenosis. This murmur is usually best heard in the left lateral position. (*10, p 1313*)

9.39 (B) Though a complete blood count is useful in evaluation of someone with heart disease, the other tests are much more important in the evaluation of the patient with valvular heart disease. (*10, pp 1313–1314, 1319*)

9.40 (B) An opening snap is associated with the first heart sound and with mitral stenosis. (*10, p 1313*)

9.41 (B) The snap or click associated with mitral valve prolapse occurs in midsystole. The murmur is a crescendo-decrescendo one in late systole. (*10, p 1317*)

9.42 (C) Severe cases of MVP may lead to mitral regurgitation rather than stenosis. (*10, p 1317*)

9.43 (B) Beta blockers are recommended for chest pain associated with MVP. (*10, p 1317*)

References

1. Joint National Committee on Prevention, Detection, Evaluation, and Treatment of High Blood Pressure: The sixth report of the Joint National Committee on Prevention, Detection, Evaluation, and Treatment of High Blood Pressure. *Arch Intern Med* 157:2413–2445, 1997.

2. http://journal.diabetes.org/fulltext/supplements/diabetescare/supplement100/s20.html.

3. McKelvie R: Heart failure. In: Godlee F (ed): *Clinical Evidence: The International Source of the Best Available Evidence for Effective Health Care,* West Allis, WI, Quad/Graphics, 2000.

4. Ferri FF: Cardiovascular diseases. In: Ferri, FF (ed): *Practical Guide to the Care of the Medical Patient,* 4/e, St. Louis, Mosby, 1998.

5. Williams GH: Hypertensive vascular disease. In: Fauci AS, Braunwald E, Isselbacher KJ, Wilson JD, Martin JB, Kasper DL, Hauser SL, Long DL (eds): *Harrison's Principles of Internal Medicine,* 14/e, New York, McGraw-Hill, 1998.

6. Creager MA, Dzau VJ: Vascular diseases of the extremities. In: Fauci AS, Braunwald E, Isselbacher KJ, Wilson JD, Martin JB, Kasper DL, Hauser SL, Long DL (eds): *Harrison's Principles of Internal Medicine,* 14/e, New York, McGraw-Hill, 1998.

7. Butler J, Braunwald E: Cor pulmonale. In: Fauci AS, Braunwald E, Isselbacher KJ, Wilson JD, Martin JB, Kasper DL, Hauser SL, Long DL (eds): *Harrison's Principles of Internal Medicine,* 14/e, New York, McGraw-Hill, 1998.

8. Bickley LS, Hoekelman RA: *Bates' Guide to Physical Examination and History Taking,* 7/e, Philadelphia, Lippincott, 1999.

9. Josephson ME, Buxton AE, Marchlinski FE: The tachy-arrhythmias. In: Fauci AS, Braunwald E, Isselbacher KJ, Wilson JD, Martin JB, Kasper DL, Hauser SL, Long DL (eds): *Harrison's Principles of Internal Medicine,* 14/e, New York, McGraw-Hill, 1998.

10. Braunwald E: Valvular heart disease. In: Fauci AS, Braunwald E, Isselbacher KJ, Wilson JD, Martin JB, Kasper DL, Hauser SL, Long DL (eds): *Harrison's Principles of Internal Medicine,* 14/e, New York, McGraw-Hill, 1998.

10

Electrocardiography

Richard R. Rahr, EdD, PA-C
Salah Ayachi, PhD, PA-C

DIRECTIONS (Questions 10.1–10.33): Each of the numbered items or incomplete statements in this chapter is followed by answers or completions of the statement. Select the **one** lettered answer or completion that is **best** in each case.

Questions 10.1–10.3: Refer to the ECG in Fig. 10.1.

10.1 The basic rhythm is
  A. Normal sinus rhythm
  B. Sinus tachycardia
  C. Sinus bradycardia
  D. Nodal rhythm
  E. Ventricular tachycardia

10.2 The atrial abnormality involves
  A. The right atrium
  B. The left atrium
  C. Both atria

10.3 The ventricular change is hypertrophy of
  A. The right ventricle
  B. The left ventricle
  C. Both ventricles

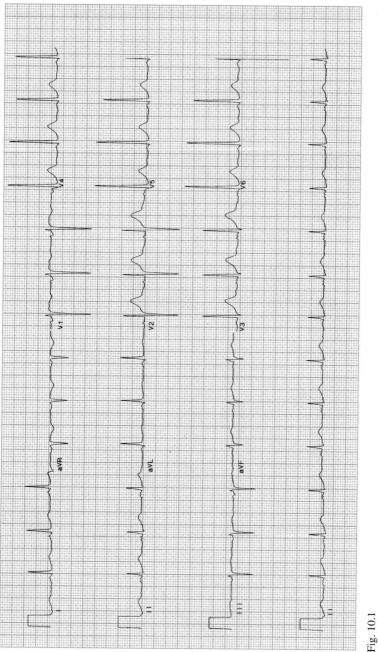

Fig. 10.1

153

Questions 10.4–10.8: Refer to the tracing in Fig. 10.2.

10.4 The basic rhythm is
  A. Normal sinus rhythm
  B. Sinus tachycardia
  C. Sinus bradycardia
  D. Ventricular tachycardia
  E. Ventricular fibrillation

10.5 What is the QRS interval?
  A. 0.08 s (80 ms)
  B. 0.16 s (160 ms)
  C. 0.12 s (120 ms)
  D. 0.36 s (360 ms)
  E. 0.20 s (200 ms)

10.6 The rate in beats per minute is
  A. 100
  B. 85
  C. 140
  D. 60
  E. 170

10.7 The conduction abnormality seen in this case is
  A. Left bundle branch block
  B. Right bundle branch block
  C. Left anterior hemiblock
  D. Right posterior hemiblock
  E. First-degree AV block

10.8 What is the correct axis in degrees?
  A. Zero
  B. +30
  C. +60
  D. −30
  E. Indeterminate

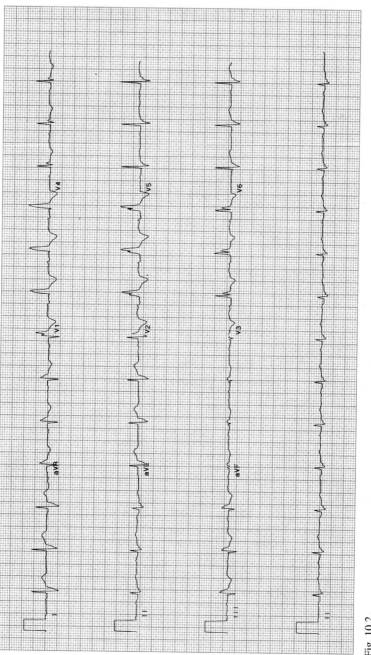

Fig. 10.2

155

Questions 10.9–10.13: Refer to the tracing in Fig. 10.3.

10.9 What is the correct axis in degrees?
  A. −30
  B. +60
  C. −60
  D. +90
  E. −90

10.10 The conduction abnormality seen here is
  A. Third-degree heart block
  B. Second-degree (Mobitz I) heart block
  C. First-degree heart block
  D. Second-degree (Mobitz II) heart block
  E. Left anterior hemiblock

10.11 The ventricular rate in beats per minute is
  A. 60
  B. 100
  C. 120
  D. 40
  E. 75

10.12 Which leads depict changes consistent with myocardial infarction?
  A. Anterior
  B. Inferior
  C. Lateral
  D. Posterior
  E. Anteroseptal

10.13 What type of conduction defect is shown?
  A. Left anterior hemiblock
  B. Left posterior hemiblock
  C. Complete right bundle branch block
  D. Incomplete left bundle branch block
  E. Third-degree heart block

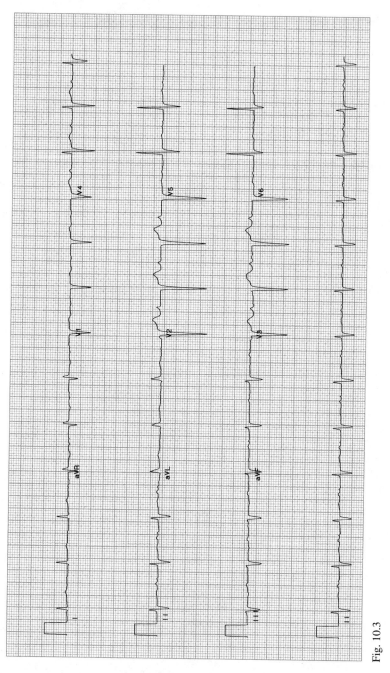

Fig. 10.3

157

Questions 10.14–10.16: Refer to the tracing in Fig. 10.4.

10.14 The rhythm is
   A. Sinus tachycardia
   B. Sinus bradycardia
   C. Normal sinus rhythm
   D. Sinus arrhythmia
   E. Ventricular tachycardia

10.15 The sum of the S in V_1 (in millimeters) and the height of the R in V_5 is greater than 35 mm in this 42-year-old woman. What is the interpretation/diagnosis?
   A. Right ventricular hypertrophy
   B. Left ventricular hypertrophy
   C. Left atrial abnormality
   D. Right atrial abnormality

10.16 The most common cause of the problem seen in question 10.15 is
   A. Hypertension
   B. Pulmonary stenosis
   C. Ventricular septal defect
   D. Atrial septal defect

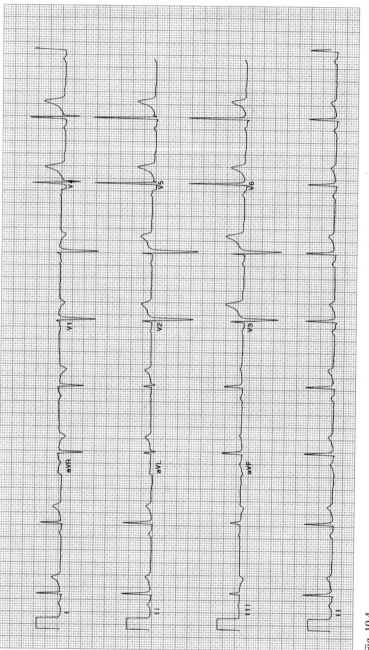

Fig. 10.4

159

Questions 10.17–10.20: Refer to the tracing in Fig. 10.5.

10.17 The P wave in leads III and AVF is peaked. This signifies
   A. Right atrial abnormality
   B. Left atrial abnormality
   C. Left ventricular hypertrophy
   D. Right ventricular hypertrophy
   E. Biatrial hypertrophy

10.18 The ventricular rate (in beats per minute) is
   A. 90
   B. 75
   C. 50
   D. 200
   E. 150

10.19 The correct axis (in degrees) in this tracing is
   A. +30
   B. Zero
   C. +15
   D. −60
   E. +90

10.20 The QRS interval in this tracing is
   A. 0.12 s (120 ms)
   B. 0.16 s (160 ms)
   C. 0.20 s (120 ms)
   D. 0.08 s (80 ms)
   E. 0.36 s (360 ms)

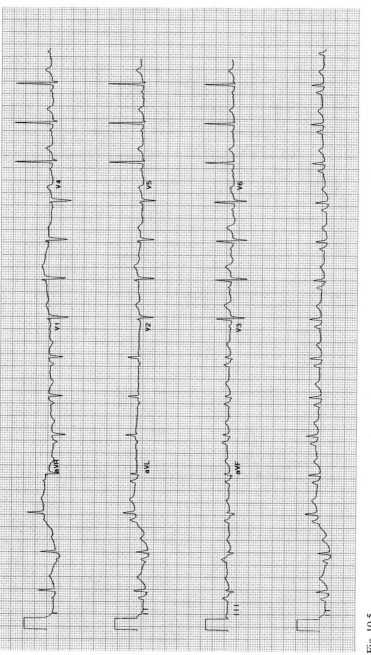

Fig. 10.5

Questions 10.21–10.24: Refer to the tracing in Fig. 10.6.

10.21 The rhythm is
   A. Sinus tachycardia
   B. Sinus arrhythmia
   C. Normal sinus rhythm
   D. Nodal rhythm
   E. Idioventricular rhythm

10.22 There is a pathologic Q wave in leads II, III, and AVF. This is consistent with
   A. Inferior MI
   B. Anterior MI
   C. Lateral MI
   D. Posterior MI
   E. High lateral MI

10.23 The axis in degrees is
   A. +30
   B. Zero
   C. −30
   D. +60
   E. +90

10.24 Is there evidence of right ventricular hypertrophy in this case?
   A. Yes
   B. No
   C. Cannot determine
   D. A second tracing is needed for comparison

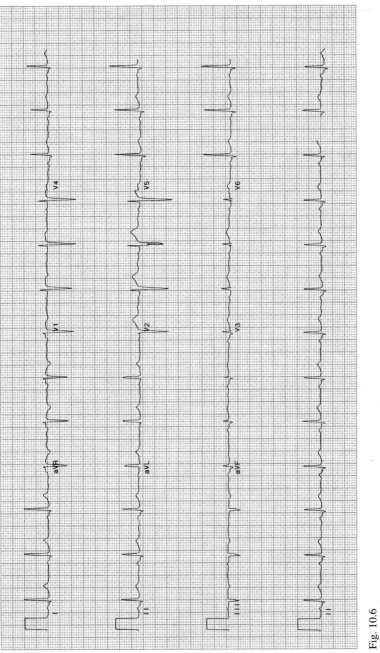

Fig. 10.6

163

Questions 10.25–10.28: Refer to the tracing in Fig. 10.7.

10.25 The tracing depicts
  A. A normal tracing
  B. An anterior MI
  C. Left ventricular hypertrophy
  D. First-degree heart block
  E. Mobitz I block

10.26 The axis in degrees is
  A. +30
  B. +150
  C. +90
  D. −120
  E. −60

10.27 The rate in beats per minute is
  A. 60
  B. 75
  C. 100
  D. 150
  E. 40

10.28 The most common arrhythmia seen in a case of acute myocardial infarction is
  A. PAC
  B. PVC
  C. Ventricular tachycardia
  D. Ventricular fibrillation

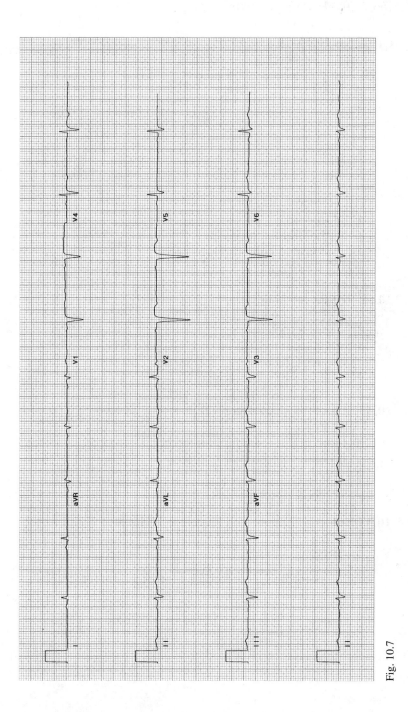

Fig. 10.7

Questions 10.29–10.33: Refer to the tracing in Fig. 10.8.

10.29 The rate in beats per minute is
  A. 60
  B. 75
  C. 100
  D. 150
  E. 200

10.30 The rhythm is
  A. Normal sinus rhythm
  B. Atrial flutter
  C. Atrial fibrillation
  D. Supraventricular tachycardia
  E. Nodal rhythm

10.31 The PR interval is
  A. 0.12 s (120 ms)
  B. 0.16 s (160 ms)
  C. 0.20 s (200 ms)
  D. 0.36 s (360 ms)
  E. Indeterminate (no P wave)

10.32 The QRS axis in degrees is
  A. +30
  B. +60
  C. −30
  D. −60
  E. +90

10.33 This tracing depicts right atrial hypertrophy.
  A. True
  B. False
  C. Indeterminate (no P wave)

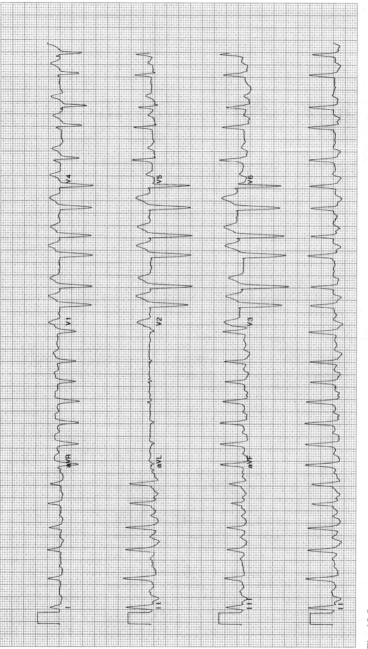

Fig. 10.8

Electrocardiography

Answers and Discussion

10.1 (A) When the P wave precedes every QRS complex, the rhythm is said to be sinus. The rate is normally 60 to 100 beats per minute (bpm). (*1, p 44*)

10.2 (B) The criterion for left atrial abnormality is a P wave in lead II that spans 0.11 s or more, or an M-shaped wave (with the spikes of the M spanning 0.04 s), or a diphasic P in lead V_1 with the negative portion spanning 0.04 s and 1 mm in depth. (*2, pp 58–60*)

10.3 (B) Using the Sokolow (voltage) method for LVH, when the sum of the S wave in V_1 and the R wave in V_5 or V_6 (whichever is larger) is greater than or equal to 35 mm, LVH is present in a patient over 30 years of age. (*2, pp 68–73*)

10.4 (A) When a P wave precedes each QRS complex, there is sinoatrial node rhythm. The rate is normally 60 to 100 bpm. (*1, p 44*)

10.5 (C) A normal QRS is 0.04 to 0.099 s long; when a QRS spans 0.10 s or longer, there is either an incomplete or complete bundle branch block. The QRS is wider than normal when there is an anterior or posterior hemiblock. (*1, pp 25–26, 29–31*)

10.6 (B) The rate for a regular rhythm is 300 divided by the number of dark lines (0.20 s apart) between the QRSs in lead II. Lead II is considered the universal rhythm strip. (*2, p 37*)

10.7 (B) A complete right bundle branch block (c-RBBB) is diagnosed when the QRS spans 0.12 s or longer (as determined on lead II), an RSR' pattern is seen in V_1, and a wide S is seen in leads I and V_6. The wide QRS, hallmark of RBBB, is such because of asynchronous ventricular depolarization that results in splitting of the depolarization wave. (*2, p 86–87*)

10.8 (E) The smallest and/or equiphasic lead is AVF, but lead I is negative (below the baseline). All limb leads are equiphasic, making the axis indeterminate. If lead I were positive (upright), the axis would be zero. (*1, pp 221–226*)

10.9 (C) The smallest and/or equiphasic lead is AVR, with lead I being upright or positive. This makes the axis −60°. (*1, pp 221–226*)

10.10 (C) First-degree AV block is diagnosed when the PR interval in lead II is over 0.20 s (200 ms). (*1, pp 143–145*)

10.11 (E) The rate is determined by dividing the number of bold lines separating QRS complexes into 300 (i.e., 300/4 = 75 bpm). (*1, pp 26–27*)

10.12 (E) There is a QS (i.e., Q wave) complex in leads V_1–V_3, which is consistent with the definition of an anteroseptal myocardial infarction. (*3, pp 83–86*)

10.13 (A) The criteria for left anterior hemiblock (LAH) are (1) a small Q in lead I, (2) left axis deviation (axis = −60°), and (3) wide S waves in leads II, III, and AVF. (*1, p 219*)

10.14 (B) Sinus bradycardia is a normal sinus rhythm (upright P in lead II) at a rate below 60 bpm. (*1, pp 46–49*)

10.15 (B) See answer 10.3.

10.16 (A) Long-standing (secondary, essential, or malignant) hypertension often causes left ventricular hypertrophy and volume overload. (*2, p 61*)

10.17 (A) The criterion for right atrial abnormality is a peaked (2.5 mm or taller) P wave in leads II, III, and AVF. This is usually associated with pulmonary disease and cor pulmonale. (*2, p 61*)

10.18 (A) The rate is 90 to 95 bpm. (*2, p 37*)

10.19 (A) The smallest or equiphasic lead is lead III; with lead I being upright or positive, the axis is +30°. (*1, pp 221–226*)

10.20 (D) The QRS interval is two boxes (0.04 s × 2) wide or 0.08 s (80 ms). (*1, pp 29–30*)

10.21 (C) It is normal sinus rhythm when the P wave is upright in lead II and the rate is 60 to 100 bpm. (*1, p 44*)

10.22 (A) There is a pathologic Q wave (0.04 s wide, or 25% of the height of the R wave) in leads II, III, and AVF; this is consistent with inferior myocardial infarction. (*3, pp 80–81*)

10.23 (B) Lead AVF is the smallest and/or most equiphasic and lead I is upright; this makes for an axis of zero. (*1, pp 221–226*)

10.24 (B) There is no RVH because the R wave in V_1 is not 7 mm tall and the R:S ratio is not equal to or greater than 1.0. (*3, pp 160–161*)

10.25 (B) The wide and deep pathologic Q waves in leads V_1–V_3 mean that there is an anterior myocardial infarction of undetermined age. (*3, pp 75–86*)

10.26 (E) The smallest and/or equiphasic lead is AVR, and lead I is upright; this makes for an axis of −60° or LAD. (*1, pp 221–226*)

10.27 (A) The sinus rate is 60 bpm. (*2, p 37*)

10.28 (B) Premature ventricular contractions are the most common arrhythmias or ectopic beats that accompany myocardial infarctions. (*3, p 82*)

10.29 (D) The rate is 150 bpm. Both rate and rhythm are irregularly irregular; this is pathognomonic of atrial fibrillation. The rate must be determined using the 6-s strip method. (*2, pp 95–100*)

10.30 (C) The rhythm is ectopic and irregular; this is consistent with atrial fibrillation. (*1, pp 95–100*)

10.31 (E) The PR interval is impossible to calculate because the P waves are nondiscernible in atrial fibrillation. (*1, pp 95–100*)

10.32 (B) The AVL lead is the smallest and/or equiphasic, and lead I is upright; this makes for an axis of +60°. (*1, pp 221–226*)

10.33 (C) No discernible P waves are found with atrial fibrillation; therefore right atrial hypertrophy cannot be diagnosed. (*1, pp 95–100*)

References

1. Lewis KM: *Sensible ECG Analysis,* Albany, NY, Delmar, 2000.

2. Wagner GS: *Marriott's Practical Electrocardiography,* 9/e, Baltimore, Williams & Wilkins, 1994.

3. Constant J: *Essentials of Learning Electrocardiography,* New York, Parthenon, 1997.

11

Neurology

Charles Haney, PA-C
Amy McAlister, PA-C

DIRECTIONS (Questions: 11.1–11.20): Each of the numbered items or incomplete statements in this chapter is followed by answers or completions of the statement. Select the **one** lettered answer or completion that is **best** in each case.

11.1 A patient with a Glasgow Coma Scale score of 3 has the following exam
   A. Eyes open spontaneously; withdraws to pain; mumbles incomprehensibly
   B. Eyes open to stimulus; follows commands in all extremities; intubated
   C. Eyes closed; no response to pain; no vocalization
   D. Eyes closed; extensor posturing in upper extremities; mumbles incomprehensibly

11.2 The most common site of origin for emboli causing ischemic stroke is the
   A. Vertebral artery
   B. Common carotid bifurcation
   C. Aortic arch
   D. Atrium

11.3 A patient with a complete left homonymous hemianopsia is most likely to have a lesion in the
   A. Right frontal lobe
   B. Right occipital lobe
   C. Left occipital lobe
   D. Left parietal lobe

11.4 The most common cause of subarachnoid hemorrhage is
   A. Head trauma
   B. Rupture of cerebral aneurysm
   C. Brain tumor
   D. Arteriovenous malformation

11.5 The most common central nervous system tumor is
   A. Glioblastoma multiforme
   B. Schwannoma
   C. Meningioma
   D. Secondary metastasis

11.6 The most common cause of new-onset seizures in a patient over age 50 is
   A. Acute infection
   B. Cerebrovascular disease
   C. Brain tumors
   D. Congenital malformation

11.7 The most common cause of defective cerebral development in industrialized nations is
   A. Advanced maternal age
   B. Fetal alcohol syndrome
   C. Single gene defects
   D. Intrauterine infections

11.8 The most common cause of bacterial meningitis in neonates is
   A. *Haemophilus influenzae*
   B. Staphylococci
   C. Gram-negative bacilli
   D. *Streptococcus pneumoniae*

11.9 The most common clinical manifestation in a patient with a brain abscess is

A. Headache
B. Fever
C. Seizure
D. Focal neurologic deficit

11.10 Treatment of Wernicke-Korsakoff syndrome includes
A. Phenobarbital
B. Phenytoin
C. Thiamine
D. Calcium channel blockers

11.11 A 42-year-old Hispanic man was injured at work when a large pipe fell on him. He presents with back pain radiating into both legs, numbness in the buttocks and posterior legs, 4/5 strength in left plantar flexion, and absent ankle reflexes. Postvoid residual volume is 1200 ml. You strongly suspect
A. Left L_4 radiculopathy
B. Brown-Sequard syndrome
C. Central cord syndrome
D. Cauda equina syndrome

11.12 A 12-year-old girl involved in a high-speed motor accident presents with a Glasgow Coma Scale score of 7. She has been intubated due to respiratory distress. Her right pupil is 8 mm and nonreactive, and her left pupil is 3 mm and reactive. She localizes with the left arm, but demonstrates flexor posturing with the right arm. CT of her brain most likely will show
A. Aneurysm
B. Hydrocephalus
C. Left subdural hematoma
D. Right epidural hematoma

11.13 A 56-year-old nurse complains of a 2-day history of severe burning pain on the left side of her face involving the forehead. She does not recall any trauma or insect bites, but has started to notice a few erythematous lesions in this region as well. You prepare to
A. Prescribe famciclovir
B. Refer to ophthalmology
C. Prescribe prednisone
D. Do all of the above

11.14 A 75-year-old man is referred to you for low back pain. Upon questioning him, you realize the pain is mostly in his legs, and he experiences it only when he walks. He must stop and rest after about 100 ft or bend forward at the waist to get relief. He has good strength in his lower extremities and sensation is intact. His lumbar spine MRI most likely shows
 A. An epidural abscess
 B. Lumbar stenosis
 C. Herniated L_5–S_1 disc
 D. Spondyloesthesis

11.15 A woman has a seizure disorder characterized by a feeling of anxiousness and nausea followed by a lapse of consciousness that lasts about 1 min. Her mother says the woman's right arm typically shows repetitive movements during her seizures. These seizures are classified as
 A. Complex partial seizures
 B. Generalized convulsive seizures
 C. Simple partial seizures
 D. None of the above

11.16 A known seizure patient arrives to your clinic complaining of gait disturbance and new-onset diplopia. Several weeks ago the patient's wife noticed "jerky eye movements" when the patient looked to the side. The most likely diagnosis is
 A. Simple partial seizures
 B. Phenytoin toxicity
 C. Brain tumor
 D. Subarachnoid hemorrhage

11.17 A 35-year-old man with a known history of psychosis controlled with haloperidol is seen in the emergency department with progressive rigidity, tremors, and postural instability. The most likely diagnosis is
 A. Depression
 B. Myasthenia gravis
 C. Alzheimer's disease
 D. Drug-induced Parkinson's disease

11.18 A 35-year-old woman presents with visual field defects and complains of not having had her period for 6 mo. She also reports new onset of breast milk even though her last child was born 5 years earlier. The most likely diagnosis is
   A. Pregnancy
   B. Ovarian cancer
   C. Pituitary tumor
   D. Cushing's syndrome

11.19 A patient presents to the emergency department after falling and hitting his head. He reports only minor headache, but is unable to open his left eye. Upon examination, the left pupil is noted to be 8 mm and nonreactive, and the right pupil is 3 mm and reactive. CT of the brain is negative. The patient has suffered an injury to cranial nerve
   A. V
   B. VII
   C. II
   D. III

11.20 A man in his forties presents to the ER complaining of the "worst headache of my life" that began about 7 h earlier. The headache began acutely and has not lessened despite OTC analgesics. CT scan is negative. Lumbar puncture results demonstrate xanthochromia of the CSF. Your diagnosis is
   A. Subarachnoid hemorrhage
   B. Epidural hematoma
   C. Bacterial meningitis
   D. Viral meningitis

Neurology

Answers and Discussion

11.1 (C)   A Glasgow Coma Scale score of 3 or 4 is correlated with an 85% chance of the patient dying or remaining vegetative, while scores above 11 indicate a 5% to 10% likelihood of death or vegetative state and an 85% chance of moderate disability or good recovery. Intermediate scores correlate with proportional chances of patients recovering. (*1, p 2396*)

11.2 (B)   The origin of the internal carotid artery is the most common site of atherosclerosis and thrombosis that leads to stroke or transient ischemic attacks. The aortic arch and atrium are occasionally associated. (*1, p 2328*)

11.3 (B)   Homonymous hemianopsia is a visual field defect affecting the right or left halves of both eyes. A left homonymous hemianopsia would arise from damage to the right optic tract or the right occipital lobe. (*1, p 163*)

11.4 (B)   Subarachnoid hemorrhage is most commonly caused by rupture of an intracranial aneurysm; arteriovenous malformation is the second most common cause. Approximately 20% of subarachnoid hemorrhages are of unknown etiology. (*1, pp 2345–2347*)

11.5 (D)   The most common central nervous system tumor is secondary metastasis. Lung, breast, melanoma, and renal tumors are the most common primaries. Gliomas are the most common CNS primary tumors, followed by meningiomas. (*1, p 2398*)

11.6 (B) The most common cause of new-onset seizures in patients older than 50 is cerebrovascular disease. Seizures can occur acutely in patients with hemorrhage or ischemic stroke. Patients with brain tumors may also present with seizures in this age group. Those with congenital malformations may present with seizures, but will do so at an early age. Infections may cause seizures at any age, especially in the young. (*1, p 2316*)

11.7 (B) The most common cause of defective cerebral development in industrial nations is fetal alcohol syndrome. Its incidence is estimated to be 1:700 live births in the U.S., much greater than that of trisomy 21 (Down syndrome) and fragile X syndrome. (*2, p 759*)

11.8 (C) Bacterial meningitis in neonates is most commonly due to gram-negative bacilli acquired in the birth canal. Gram-negative bacilli can also be seen in elderly debilitated patients. *H. influenzae* is usually seen in preschool children. *S. pneumoniae* is commonly seen in adults and elderly patients. *Staphylococcus aureus* can be seen in diabetics, and *S. aureus* pneumonia occurs in cancer patients. (*1, p 2419*)

11.9 (A) Headache is the most common clinical manifestation of brain abscess. The triad of fever, headache, and focal deficit is prevalent in greater than 50% of patients; over 70% will present with headache. Seizures occur in ~25% to 40% of patients. (*1, p 2428*)

11.10 (C) Wernicke-Korsakoff syndrome should be treated promptly with large parenteral doses of thiamine. Early manifestations of thiamine deficiency include anorexia, muscle cramps, paresthesias, and irritability. Thiamine deficiency in the U.S. is largely due to alcoholism. (*1, p 2455; 2, p 1064*)

11.11 (D) Cauda equina syndrome is characterized by radiating back pain, numbness in the buttocks, decreased strength, and urinary retention. An L_4 radiculopathy would only affect the L_4 dermatome. Brown-Sequard syndrome is a lesion involving the spinal cord extensively on one side of the midline resulting in ipsilateral motor weakness and proprioception and contralateral loss of pain perception below the injury. Central cord syndrome is produced by brief compression of the cord and disruption of the central gray matter; there is weakness of the arms, often with loss or decrease of sensation over the shoulders and arms. Lower extremity strength is usually spared, but bladder function is variable. (*1, p 2382; 3, pp 824–825*)

11.12 (D) Epidural hematomas are most commonly seen in the temporal lobes, where the skull is the thinnest and meningeal blood vessels are numerous. Fractures of the temporal bone can easily lacerate the meningeal arteries. Expansion of the hematoma causes compression of the temporal lobe that causes contralateral hemiparesis, dilation of the ipsilateral pupil, and eventual herniation. (*3, p 822*)

11.13 (D) Patients with zoster lesions involving the trigeminal nerve should always be sent to an ophthalmologist to evaluate lesions in the ophthalmic division of the trigeminal nerve. Corticosteroids have been used to reduce the incidence of postherpetic neuralgia. (*1, p 2445*)

11.14 (B) Lumbar stenosis causes intermittent and chronic compression of the cauda equina because of congenital narrowing of the lumbar spinal canal. Exercise brings on aching pain in the buttocks, thighs, and calves; the pain stops with rest. (*1, p 77*)

11.15 (A) Complex partial seizures are associated with impaired consciousness accompanied by focal motor or somatosensory symptoms. Simple partial seizures are similar but without the impaired consciousness. Generalized convulsive seizures are characterized by sudden loss of consciousness; the patient becomes rigid and respiration is arrested. This phase, the tonic phase, usually lasts less than 1 min and is followed by a clonic phase in which there is jerking of the body that can last 2 to 3 min. (*2, p 966*)

11.16 (B) Dilantin can have dose-related effects including early nystagmus, diplopia, and ataxia. The nystagmus usually requires no dose adjustment, but the diplopia and ataxia are indications for dose reduction. Gingival hyperplasia and hirsutism occur to some degree in most patients. Chronic use may affect vitamin D metabolism, leading to osteomalacia. (*4, pp 363–365*)

11.17 (D) Haloperidol blocks dopamine receptors, and therefore may produce a parkinsonian syndrome. This usually occurs within 3 mo of initial treatment, is usually dose-related, and will clear over weeks to months after discontinuation. (*4, p 427*)

11.18 (C) Pituitary tumors often cause visual field defects. This patient presents with a pituitary prolactinoma causing amenorrhea and galactorrhea. (*3, p 838*)

11.19 (D) Patients with oculomotor nerve palsy present with a dilated pupil nonreactive to light and with ptosis. Those with trigeminal nerve palsy present with weak or absent contraction of the temporal and masseter muscles. Trauma to the optic nerve results in decreased visual acuity. Facial nerve trauma affects the muscles of facial expression, impairing the patient's ability to raise the eyebrows, smile, and show the teeth. (*5, pp 217, 570, 608*)

11.20 (A) Subarachnoid hemorrhage is sometimes not visualized on CT scan, necessitating a lumbar puncture for evaluation of subarachnoid blood. Xanthochromia is caused by the breakdown of red blood cells. (*1, pp 2345–2346*)

References

1. Fauci AS, Braunwald E, Isselbacher KJ, Wilson JD, Martin JB, Kasper DL, Hauser SL, Longo DL: *Harrison's Principles of Internal Medicine,* 14/e, New York, McGraw-Hill, 1998.

2. Tierney LM, McPhee SJ, Papadakis MA: *Current Medical Diagnosis & Treatment,* 39/e, New York, McGraw-Hill, 2000.

3. Way L: *Current Surgical Diagnosis & Treatment,* 10/e, Norwalk, CT, Appleton & Lange, 1994.

4. Katzung B: *Basic and Clinical Pharmacology,* 7/e, Stamford, CT, Appleton & Lange, 1997.

5. Bickley LS, Hoekelman RA: *Bates' Guide to Physical Examination and History Taking,* 7/e, Philadelphia, Lippincott, 1997.

12

Pulmonary System

Marilyn R. Childers, MEd, RRT

DIRECTIONS (Questions 12.1–12.30): Each of the numbered items or incomplete statements in this chapter is followed by answers or completions of the statement. Select the **one** lettered answer or completion that is **best** in each case.

12.1 Laryngotracheobronchitis (aka croup) is most commonly caused by
- **A.** Mycoplasma
- **B.** *Pseudomonas aeruginosa*
- **C.** Pneumocystis
- **D.** Parainfluenza viruses

12.2 The following are blood gas results of a 34-year-old man during an asthma attack: PaO_2, 72; $PaCO_2$, 30; HCO_3^-, 25; pH, 7.50. Which of the following interpretations correctly identifies the problem?
- **A.** Chronic alveolar hyperventilation
- **B.** Acute alveolar hyperventilation
- **C.** Acute alveolar hyperventilation with hypoxemia
- **D.** Respiratory acidosis
- **E.** Respiratory alkalosis with adequate oxygenation

12.3 A diagnosis of childhood cystic fibrosis is made when the concentration of sodium chloride in the sweat is above
   A. 40 mEq/L
   B. 50 mEq/L
   C. 60 mEq/L
   D. 70 mEq/L
   E. 80 mEq/L

12.4 In which type of lung cancer is sputum **NOT** useful as a diagnostic tool?
   A. Squamous cell carcinoma
   B. Adenocarcinoma
   C. Large cell carcinoma
   D. Small cell carcinoma

12.5 Which of the following is **NOT** routinely associated with bronchogenic carcinoma?
   A. Coin lesion on chest x-ray
   B. Hoarseness
   C. Increased sputum production
   D. Cyanosis
   E. Increased chest expansion

12.6 Which condition does **NOT** produce a dull percussion note?
   A. Tension pneumothorax
   B. Pleural effusion
   C. Atelectasis
   D. Pneumonia

Questions 12.7–12.10: Match the lettered items (breath sounds) with the numbered items (descriptors).
   A. Vesicular
   B. Crackles
   C. Bronchial
   D. Stridor

12.7 Breath sounds heard over the trachea and large airways

12.8 Sounds both heard and auscultated over the trachea due to obstruction of the upper (supraglottic) airway

12.9 Breath sounds heard over the lung periphery

12.10 Airflow causing movement of excessive secretions or fluid in the airways

12.11 A hospitalized patient is diagnosed with community-acquired pneumonia. Which antibiotic(s) would you recommend for treatment of this condition?
  A. Macrolide plus a third-generation cephalosporin
  B. Tetracycline plus a carbapenem
  C. β-lactam plus a quinolone
  D. Penicillin
  E. Monobactam

12.12 Which of the following is **NOT** a common symptom of COPD?
  A. Cough
  B. Increased sputum production
  C. Dyspnea on exertion
  D. Shortness of breath
  E. Low-grade fever

12.13 Calcification along the pleural borders seen on chest x-ray suggests exposure to
  A. Asbestos
  B. Copper sulfate
  C. Polyurethane foams
  D. Pesticides
  E. Plastics

12.14 Which of the following does **NOT** produce exudative pleural effusion?
  A. Carcinoma
  B. Tuberculosis
  C. Pneumonia
  D. Systemic lupus
  E. Cirrhosis

12.15 Which of the following would be the drug of choice to treat acute bronchoconstriction and resultant airway narrowing?
  A. Salmeterol
  B. Ipratropium bromide
  C. Albuterol
  D. Intal
  E. Dexamethasone

12.16 Inhaled corticosteroids are used for long-term treatment of asthma because they
  A. Relax bronchial smooth muscle
  B. Have anti-inflammatory properties
  C. Inhibit histamine release in the lungs
  D. Block adenosine receptors in the smooth muscle of the lungs
  E. Decrease mucus production

12.17 Which of the following can decrease blood levels of theophylline?
  A. Beta blockers
  B. Cigarette smoking
  C. Corticosteroids
  D. Alcohol
  E. Cirrhosis

12.18 Surfactant replacement therapy can be used for
  A. Chronic obstructive pulmonary disease
  B. Cystic fibrosis with an upper respiratory infection
  C. Nosocomial pneumonia
  D. Respiratory distress syndrome in the neonate
  E. Sarcoidosis

12.19 A patient presents to the ER with severe carbon monoxide poisoning. Pulse oximetry indicates a saturation of 100%. The best course of action is to
  A. Do nothing, but monitor the patient
  B. Apply a HAFOE mask at 60%
  C. Use a nonrebreather mask at an appropriate flow rate
  D. Provide hyperbaric oxygen therapy

12.20 Which of the following is **NOT** usually associated with digital clubbing?
   A. Interstitial lung disease
   B. COPD
   C. Bronchiectasis
   D. Lung cancer
   E. Congenital heart defects

12.21 Which device would you order for a COPD patient with increased inspiratory demand requiring oxygen therapy at 24%?
   A. Nasal cannula
   B. Nonrebreather mask
   C. Simple mask
   D. Air entrainment mask (Ventimask)
   E. Transtracheal oxygen

12.22 Which of the following is **NOT** an indication for postural drainage therapy?
   A. Sputum production of 5 to 10 mL/day in the adult
   B. Atelectasis due to mucus plugging
   C. Retained secretions in patients with artificial airways
   D. Foreign body in the airway
   E. Cystic fibrosis

12.23 Which of the following is **NOT** a contraindication to bronchial hygiene therapy?
   A. ICP > 20 mm Hg
   B. Untreated tension pneumothorax
   C. Bronchopleural fistula
   D. Pulmonary embolism
   E. Chest tubes

12.24 A patient arrives in the emergency room with an esophageal obturator airway (EOA) in place. Which of the following is the correct procedure to follow for intubation?
   A. Suction and remove the EOA, then intubate
   B. Intubate the airway and leave the EOA in place
   C. Intubate the airway and then remove the EOA
   D. Remove the EOA and intubate the patient

12.25 Which of the following would not be an appropriate way to increase $Paco_2$ in the mechanically ventilated patient?
A. Increase the oxygen concentration
B. Decrease the tidal volume
C. Decrease the rate
D. Begin sedation

12.26 A 54-year-old, 55-kg (IBW = 54 kg) woman is being ventilated. Pertinent data is as follows: mode, SIMV; VT, 550 mL; Pao_2, 84 mm Hg; rate, 14; PEEP, +5 cm H_2O; $Paco_2$, 31 mm Hg; Fio_2, 40%; pH, 7.49. Which of the following changes would you recommend at this time?
A. Increase PEEP to 10 cm H_2O
B. Decrease Fio_2 to 30%
C. Increase VT to 800 mL
D. Decrease frequency to 10 breaths per minute

12.27 A 60-year-old, 70-kg emphysema patient is being mechanically ventilated. Pertinent data follows: mode, SIMV; V_T, 560 mL; $Paco_2$, 45 mm Hg; rate, 12; spontaneous rate, 0; HCO_3, 39 mEq/L; Fio_2, 0.75; pH, 7.38; Pao_2, 160 mm Hg. To initiate weaning the patient from the ventilator, which of the following should the care provider recommend be adjusted first?
A. Mode
B. Fio_2
C. Tidal volume
D. Rate
E. PEEP

12.28 An alert 26-year-old patient is scheduled for surgery to repair tendon and ligament damage stemming from years of competitive running. As part of the preoperative workup, the following data is gathered: Fio_2, 21%; T, 37.4°C; saturation (by pulse ox), 98%; RR, 10; Pao_2, 125 mm Hg; pulse, 45; $Paco_2$, 33 mm Hg; BP, 110/60; pH, 7.47. Which of the following should be recommended in view of this data?
A. An electrocardiogram
B. Administration of oxygen at 6 L by nasal cannula
C. Repeat arterial blood gas studies
D. Intubation and continuous mechanical ventilation

12.29 Decreased FEV_1, normal to increased FEV_1/FVC, and decreased FEF_{25-75} are consistent with
  A. Restrictive lung disease
  B. Obstructive lung disease
  C. Normal lung

12.30 A patient has performed a basic spirometry and D_LCO_{SB} (diffusion capacity test) with the following results: decreased FEV_1; decreased FEV_1/FVC; decreased FEF_{25-75}; decreased FVC; decreased TLC; decreased D_LCO_{SB}. Which of the following most accurately describes the patient's condition?
  A. Chronic bronchitis
  B. Cystic fibrosis
  C. Asthma
  D. Emphysema

Pulmonary System

Answers and Discussion

12.1 (D) Parainfluenza virus is the most common pathogen in laryngotracheobronchitis (croup) in infants aged 3 mo to 3 years. Other, less common, pathogens include influenza A and B, respiratory syncytial virus, adenovirus, and rhinovirus. Mycoplasma and pneumocystis are other pathogens that cause inflammation of the gas exchange units of the lungs. (*1, p 508*)

12.2 (C) Assessment of arterial blood gas begins with interpretation of the $Paco_2$ and pH to determine acid-base status. In this case, $Paco_2$ is decreased (due to hyperventilation) and pH · is elevated; this is consistent with acute respiratory alkalosis, given the patient's condition and the fact that the HCO_3^- level is normal. Lastly, the probable cause of the respiratory alkalosis is either hypoxemia or respiratory center stimulation, with hypoxemia being more likely in this case. (*2, p 73*)

12.3 (C) A sweat chloride level of over 60 mEq/L is diagnostic of cystic fibrosis in a child. This test is not necessarily diagnostic in adults because of the higher electrolyte content of sweat in adults. (*3, p 170*)

12.4 (D) The usefulness of cytologic examination of sputum for detection of small cell carcinoma (SCC) is limited because

190

SCCs are located in the submucosa. Cytologic examination can be up to 90% accurate in detecting squamous cell carcinoma. (*3, p 258*)

12.5 (E)   In bronchogenic carcinoma, lung volumes and capacities are often decreased, leading to reduced chest expansion. Lung expansion can be further decreased due to decreased lung compliance. (*2, pp 233–234*)

12.6 (A)   Percussion notes are dull over areas of pleural thickening, atelectasis, or consolidation because of lack of air in these areas. The notes are hyperresonant over areas of increased air trapping. (*1, p 8*)

12.7–12.10 (C); (D); (A); (B)   Bronchial breath sounds are normally heard over the trachea and larger airways. They are characterized by their high pitch and loudness. Stridor is often audible and is due to rapid gas flow through a narrowed supraglottic airway. Stridor is usually high-pitched and monophonic (sounding like a single note). Vesicular breath sounds are normal breath sounds heard over the lung periphery. Crackles can be heard when airflow causes movement of secretions; these can often be cleared after a patient produces an effective cough. Crackles can also be heard when collapsed airways are reopened during inspiration. (*4, pp 313–314*)

12.11 (A)   According to the American Thoracic Society, hospitalized patients with community-acquired pneumonia should be treated with a macrolide plus a second- or third-generation cephalosporin or a β-lactam/β-lactamase inhibitor. (*4, p 436*)

12.12 (E)   Low-grade fever is usually seen with a respiratory infection and is not part of the normal symptoms of the COPD patient. Due to increased sputum production, COPD patients often have a chronic cough. Shortness of breath is related to hypoxemia, and is exacerbated during exertion. (*4, p 444*)

12.13 (A)   Calcification is often seen along the pleura in the chest x-ray of a patient with a history of asbestos exposure. This calcification may not cause symptoms or physiologic abnormalities, but can provide additional information for the diagnosis of asbestos exposure in interstitial lung disease. (*4, p 467*)

12.14 (E) Exudative pleural effusions are caused by inflammation of the pleura or lungs. Transudative pleural effusions are seen when there has been no damage to the pleura. Carcinoma, tuberculosis, pneumonia, and systemic lupus all can cause inflammation of the pleura or lungs resulting in exudative effusion. Transudative effusions account for about 70% of pleural effusions and are commonly caused by congestive heart failure, cirrhosis, and atelectasis. (*4, pp 477–479*)

12.15 (C) Albuterol is a rapidly acting β-adrenergic agonist used to treat bronchoconstriction during the acute phase. It has an onset of action of 4 to 6 min and peaks in about 60 min, with duration of action of 4 to 6 h. Salmeterol is a long-acting β-adrenergic agonist used for maintenance therapy. Ipratropium bromide is an anticholinergic agent used for long-term maintenance therapy of the COPD patient. Intal is a mediator-modifying agent used prophylactically to prevent the onset of bronchoconstriction. Lastly, dexamethasone, a corticosteroid used via the inhaled route, is used as a long-term anti-inflammatory, but is not appropriate for acute situations. (*3, p 109*)

12.16 (B) Corticosteroids, either intravenous or inhaled, work through several mechanisms to decrease inflammation in the lungs. In general, corticosteroids increase anti-inflammatory proteins and decrease proinflammatory proteins at the cellular level. (*5, p 196*)

12.17 (C) Theophylline is metabolized by the liver and excreted by the kidneys. Therefore, any disease state or drug that affects liver and kidney function will potentially affect theophylline levels in the body. Cigarette smoking stimulates liver enzymes that deactivate methylanxines, including theophylline. (*5, p 148*)

12.18 (D) Surfactant replacement therapy is designed to replenish surfactant levels in neonates with respiratory distress syndrome (RDS). The indications are treatment of infants with birth weights under 1350 g, prophylactic use in infants under 1350 g who show signs of RDS, and treatment of infants who have developed RDS. (*3, p 185*)

12.19 (D) Patients with carbon monoxide poisoning routinely have saturations of 100% by pulse oximetry. Since the pulse oximeter measures only bound hemoglobin and does not distinguish between oxygen and carbon dioxide, it becomes unreliable in a clinical situation of this type. Additional testing can be done with an arterial blood gas and a cooximeter; the latter measures carbon monoxide levels. In the situation described, it is imperative that carbon monoxide be displaced from the hemoglobin as quickly as possible. The best way to achieve this is with the highest Fio_2 available, which can be achieved in hyperbaric chambers. (*4, pp 361, 764*)

12.20 (B) Digital clubbing is usually not seen in patients with asthma or COPD. Although the specific cause is unknown, the following factors may be involved: (1) circulating vasodilators, (2) chronic infection, (3) toxins, (4) capillary stasis, (5) arterial hypoxia, and (6) local hypoxia. Clubbing is seen in a number of conditions including interstitial lung disease, bronchiectasis, various cancers, congenital heart defects (causing cyanosis), inflammatory bowel disease, and chronic liver disease. (*1, p 70; 4, pp 317–318*)

12.21 (D) Patients with COPD rely on their elevated CO_2 levels and on the hypoxic drive sensed by the peripheral chemoreceptors. Giving these patients too high an oxygen concentration suppresses their hypoxic drive and causes hypoventilation. In most cases, for the alert patient with COPD, it is important to provide high levels of gas flow with a low, precise oxygen concentration. The AEM (air entrainment mask) is ideally suited for this patient. Due to the high flows achieved with these masks, there is less room air inhaled during the respiratory cycle, therefore maintaining a more precise oxygen concentration. Also, at low oxygen concentrations, flows can reach up to 100 L/min or more, meeting the patient's increased inspiratory demands. The nasal cannula, simple mask, nonrebreather mask, and transtracheal oxygen are all low-flow systems that will not meet the patient's inspiratory demands. (*4, pp 742–755*)

12.22 (A) Postural drainage is used to position the patient to allow gravity to help move secretions from distal areas of the lungs to more centrally located airways and permit expectoration. Therefore, patients who have difficulty removing secretions will benefit from postural drainage therapy. Sputum production is a normal process of the tracheobronchial tree; usually, not enough sputum is produced to require postural drainage therapy. If the patient is having difficulty clearing secretions and is producing an excessive amount of secretions (>25 to 30 mL/day), postural drainage therapy is indicated. (*6, p 1419*)

12.23 (E) Chest tubes do not pose a problem when postural drainage and percussion therapy are being used, provided measures are taken to not dislodge the tubes during positioning and to avoid percussion over the tube site. According to the AARC Clinical Practice Guideline, positioning patients for bronchial hygiene therapy is contraindicated in numerous conditions, including unstable head and neck injuries, active hemorrhage with hemodynamic instability, elevated intracranial pressure, recent spinal surgery, active hemoptysis, empyema, bronchopleural fistula, and others. (*6, p 1419*)

12.24 (C) Esophageal obturator airways (EOAs) may be used by untrained personnel to establish an airway during an emergency procedure. Since the EOA is inserted into the esophagus, its removal will often cause vomiting, which may lead to aspiration. For this reason, it is imperative that intubation take place prior to removal of the EOA. (*7, pp 160–161*)

12.25 (A) To increase the $Paco_2$ via the pulmonary system, a reduction in alveolar ventilation is needed. Decreasing the tidal volume and respiratory rate would decrease alveolar ventilation and increase the $Paco_2$ level. Sedation would reduce the respiratory center drive and decrease alveolar ventilation. Increasing the oxygen concentration would alter the Pao_2, but would not affect the $Paco_2$ level directly. (*4, pp 909–911*)

12.26 (D) The patient is exhibiting respiratory alkalosis due to hyperventilation. Since the tidal volume is adequate at 10 mL/kg, it would be most beneficial to decrease the rate at this time to reduce alveolar ventilation, thereby increasing the $Paco_2$. Adjusting the PEEP would affect oxygenation and possibly the hemodynamic status, whereas altering the Fio_2 would affect the Pao_2. (*4, pp 909–911*)

12.27 (B) When the weaning process is begun, the patient should be spontaneously breathing to some degree. In this case, the spontaneous rate is zero and the patient is being fully supported by the mechanical ventilator. Since the patient has emphysema, you should remember that the drive to breathe is due to low oxygen levels detected by peripheral chemoreceptors and elevated $Paco_2$ levels. In this case, because the oxygen concentration is too high, the acid-base status must be returned to baseline before weaning can take place. This can be done by lowering the oxygen concentration and allowing the patient's $Paco_2$ to climb. (*4, pp 971–974*)

12.28 (C) This patient is an otherwise healthy individual breathing room air. Saturation (by pulse oximetry) is at 98%. The current blood gases indicate respiratory alkalosis with increased oxygen levels on room air. Arterial blood gas samples that have bubbles in them will give erroneous results. The air bubble will decrease the $Paco_2$, increase the pH, and increase the Pao_2. It is important to always review the blood gases with the patient's clinical picture to ensure adequate sampling and analysis. (*2, p 311*)

12.29 (A) Restrictive disease processes limit lung expansion, thus reducing the volume of gas that can be exhaled. Airway obstruction and resulting hyperinflation also reduce the volume of gas that can be exhaled. To differentiate the two disease processes, the FEV_1-to-FVC ratio is determined. An FEV_1/FVC of less than 70% indicates obstructive disease. Patients with restrictive disease (due to lung stiffness) have FEV_1/FVC above 70%, which is consistent with normal or increased FEV_1 and decreased FVC. (*4, p 394*)

12.30 (E) The data provided is consistent with an obstructive disease process; the patient's exhaled volumes and capacities are decreased. The diffusion capacity determines the amount of carbon monoxide that crosses the alveolar capillary membrane. In the case of emphysema, there is destruction of the alveolar capillary membrane, thereby reducing the diffusion of carbon monoxide across the membrane. (*4, p 392*)

References

1. Des Jardins T: *Clinical Manifestations of Respiratory Disease,* 2/e, Saint Louis, Year Book, 1990.

2. Shapiro BA, Peruzzi WT, Templin R: *Clinical Application of Blood Gases,* 5/e, Saint Louis, Mosby, 1994.

3. Farzan, S: *A Concise Handbook of Respiratory Diseases,* 3/e, Norwalk, CT, Appleton & Lange, 1992.

4. Scanlan CL, Wilkins RL, Stoller JK: *Egan's Fundamentals of Respiratory Care,* 7/e, Saint Louis, Mosby, 1999.

5. Rau JL: *Respiratory Care Pharmacology,* 5/e, Saint Louis, Mosby, 1998.

6. AARC Clinical Practice Guideline: Postural Drainage Therapy. *Respir Care* 36:1418–1426, 1991.

7. Branson RD, Hess DR, Chaburn RI: *Respiratory Care Equipment,* 2/e, Philadelphia, Lippincott, 1999.

13

Infectious Diseases

Roberto Canales, MS, PA-C

DIRECTIONS (Questions 13.1–13.30): Each of the numbered items or incomplete statements in this chapter is followed by answers or completions of the statement. Select the **one** lettered answer or completion that is **best** in each case.

13.1 A 5-year-old child presents with a 1-wk history of epistaxis, gingival bleeding, and multiple joint pain. Physical examination demonstrates paleness, petechiae, and hepato-splenomegaly. Which of the following is the most likely diagnosis?
   A. Acute lymphoblastic leukemia
   B. Acute myelogenous leukemia
   C. Acute nonlymphocytic leukemia
   D. Chronic lymphocytic leukemia

13.2 Which of the following is the most common AIDS-defining illness?
   A. Central nervous system toxoplasmosis
   B. *Pneumocystis carinii* pneumonia
   C. Cryptococcal meningitis
   D. Progressive multifocal leukoencephalopathy

13.3 A 36-year-old patient presents with a new diagnosis of AIDS, a nonproductive cough associated with low-grade fever, and dyspnea on exertion for the last 3 wk. Chest x-ray findings are not significant. Which of the following is the most likely diagnosis?
  A. *P. carinii* pneumonia
  B. Pulmonary tuberculosis
  C. Pulmonary histoplasmosis
  D. Cytomegalovirus (CMV) pneumonitis

13.4 At what absolute CD4 cell count can a diagnosis of AIDS be made in someone with asymptomatic HIV infection?
  A. 299 per cubic millimeter
  B. 499 per cubic millimeter
  C. 199 per cubic millimeter
  D. 399 per cubic millimeter

13.5 A 40-year-old man presents with fever, headache, and emesis. Physical exam demonstrates positive Kernig and Brudzinski signs and a petechial rash. What is the most likely diagnosis?
  A. Meningococcal meningitis
  B. Haemophilus meningitis
  C. Cryptococcal meningitis
  D. Central nervous system toxoplasmosis

13.6 Which of the following organisms is the most likely cause of an early infection following a dog or cat bite?
  A. *Pseudomonas aeruginosa*
  B. Haemophilus
  C. *Pasteurella multocida*
  D. *Staphylococcus aureus*

13.7 Which of the following is the most likely cause of nongonococcal urethritis?
  A. *Chlamydia trachomatis*
  B. *Neisseria gonorrhoeae*
  C. *Trichomonas vaginalis*
  D. *Candida albicans*

13.8 Which organism is the most common cause of native valve endocarditis?
    A. *Streptococcus viridans*
    B. *S. aureus*
    C. Klebsiella
    D. *C. albicans*

13.9 Which organism is the most common cause of native valve endocarditis in intravenous drug users?
    A. *S. viridans*
    B. *S. aureus*
    C. Klebsiella
    D. *C. albicans*

13.10 Which of the following diagnostic studies is the single most important for the diagnosis of infective endocarditis?
    A. Chest x-ray
    B. Complete blood count
    C. Blood culture
    D. Electrocardiogram

13.11 Which of the following is **NOT** considered to be one of the human herpes viruses?
    A. Varicella zoster
    B. Epstein-Barr virus
    C. Cytomegalovirus
    D. Toxoplasmosis

13.12 The prodrome of fever, coryza, cough, conjunctivitis, photophobia, and Koplik spots is most likely to be associated with which of the following?
    A. Rubella
    B. Poliomyelitis
    C. Measles
    D. Mumps

13.13 Which of the following regarding respiratory syncytial virus (RSV) is **FALSE**?
    A. It may cause pneumonia, bronchiolitis, and tracheobronchitis
    B. Rapid diagnosis may be made by using an ELISA or immunofluorescent assay.

C. Hyperimmune RSV immunoglobulin G may be given as prophylaxis.
D. Reinfection with RSV is not possible.

13.14 Which of the following is the causative agent for Rocky Mountain spotted fever?
A. *Rickettsia rickettsii*
B. *Dermacentor andersoni*
C. *Dermacentor variabilis*
D. *Rickettsia akari*

13.15 An 8-year-old presents with a painful facial lesion. Physical exam reveals a well-demarcated, tender, edematous, hot, and erythematous area and an oral temperature of 102°F. Which of the following is the most likely cause?
A. β-hemolytic streptococci
B. *S. aureus*
C. *Staphylococcus haemolyticus*
D. Group A streptococci

13.16 *Clostridium perfringens* is associated with which clinical condition?
A. Gas gangrene
B. Toxic shock syndrome
C. Botulism
D. Anthrax

13.17 Acute diarrhea with blood, fever, and crampy abdominal pain is most closely associated with which of the following?
A. *S. aureus*
B. Shigellosis
C. Crohn's disease
D. Giardiasis

13.18 Which of the following is the treatment of choice for uncomplicated gonococcal infection?
A. Ceftriaxone
B. Doxycycline
C. Amoxicillin
D. Bactrim

13.19 Chancroid is a sexually transmitted disease caused by which of the following organisms?
A. *Calymmatobacterium granulomatis*
B. Herpes simplex virus
C. *Haemophilus ducreyi*
D. *C. trachomatis*

13.20 Atypical mycobacteria include all of the following **EXCEPT**
A. *Mycobacterium tuberculosis*
B. *Mycobacterium fortuitum*
C. *Mycobacterium kansasii*
D. *Mycobacterium marinum*

13.21 Which of the following statements is **FALSE** regarding *C. trachomatis?*
A. Lymphogranuloma venereum (LGV) is an acute and chronic sexually transmitted disease caused by *C. trachomatis.*
B. A positive complement fixation test assists in the diagnosis.
C. *C. trachomatis* is probably the leading cause of infertility in females in the United States.
D. Lymph node enlargement is rare.

13.22 Which of the following sentences is **FALSE** regarding *Treponema pallidum?*
A. The fluorescent treponemal antibody absorption (FTA-ABS) test is often used in diagnosis.
B. A positive CSF VDRL may be associated with neurosyphilis.
C. Ceftriaxone is the drug of choice for treatment.
D. It is associated with a painless genital ulcer.

13.23 Primary syphilis is most associated with all of the following **EXCEPT**
A. Painless ulcer
B. Nontender enlargement of regional lymph nodes
C. Lesion occurring 2 to 6 wk after exposure
D. Generalized maculopapular skin rash

13.24 Late (tertiary) syphilis is characterized by all of the following **EXCEPT**
A. Infiltrative tumors of skin, bones, and liver (gummas)
B. Aortitis, aneurysms, and aortic regurgitation
C. Central nervous system disorders
D. Meningitis, hepatitis, osteitis, and iritis

13.25 Lyme disease is caused by which of the following?
A. *Borrelia burgdorferi*
B. *Leptospira interrogans*
C. *Leptospira autumnalis*
D. *Trypanosoma brucei rhodesiense*

13.26 Which of the following statements is **FALSE** regarding amebiasis?
A. It is caused by the protozoan *Entamoeba histolytica*.
B. Hepatic amebiasis may be a complication.
C. Transmission generally occurs through ingestion of cysts from fecally contaminated food or water.
D. It is a self-limited condition treated with supportive care.

13.27 Which of the following statements best describes giardiasis?
A. Most infections are symptomatic.
B. Cysts and occasionally trophozoites in the stool are rare.
C. Blood and pus are present in the stool.
D. It is characterized by mild to severe acute or chronic diarrhea that is greasy, frothy, and malodorous.

13.28 Which clinical condition is caused by *Taenia saginata, Taenia solium,* and *Diphyllobothrium latum?*
A. Pinworm infection
B. Tapeworm infection
C. Hookworm disease
D. Visceral larva migrans

13.29 Which clinical condition is caused by *Enterobium vermicularis,* has humans as the only host, and is associated with nocturnal perianal and vulvar pruritus?
  A. Pinworm infection
  B. Tapeworm infection
  C. Hookworm disease
  D. Visceral larva migrans

13.30 Which clinical condition is widespread in the moist tropics and subtropics and is caused by *Ancylostoma duodenale* and *Necator americanus?*
  A. Pinworm infection
  B. Tapeworm infection
  C. Hookworm disease
  D. Visceral larva migrans

Infectious Diseases

Answers and Discussion

13.1 (A) Acute lymphoblastic leukemia (ALL) comprises 80% of the acute leukemias of childhood. The peak incidence is between 3 and 7 years of age. (*1, p 506*)

13.2 (B) PCP occurs in up to 80% of patients with AIDS who are not on PCP prophylaxis. (*1, p 1392*)

13.3 (A) PCP occurs in up to 80% of patients with AIDS who are not on PCP prophylaxis. Additionally, weight loss is not mentioned; this would imply pulmonary tuberculosis. (*1, p 1392*)

13.4 (C) In 1993, the Centers for Disease Control and Prevention expanded the AIDS definition to include those with CD4 counts below 200 per cubic millimeter. (*1, p 1204*)

13.5 (A) Meningococcal meningitis is diagnosed based on the following: fever, headache, vomiting, confusion, delirium, convulsions, petechial rash of skin and mucous membranes, neck and back stiffness with positive Kernig and Brudzinski signs (characteristic), purulent spinal fluid with gram-negative intracellular and extracellular diplococci, culture of cerebrospinal fluid, blood, or petechial aspiration (confirms the diagnosis). (*1, p 1280*)

13.6 (C) The bacteriology of bite infections depends on the biting animal and when the infection occurs after the biting incident. Early infections (within 24 h after the bite) following dog and cat bites are most frequently caused by *P. multocida.* (*1, p 1189*)

13.7 (A) *C. trachomatis* immunotypes D–K are isolated in about 50% of cases of nongonococcal urethritis and cervicitis by appropriate techniques. (*1, p 1302*)

13.8 (A) Approximately 90% of cases of native valve endocarditis are due to *S. viridans* (60%), *S. aureus* (20%), and enterococci (5% to 10%). Gram-negative organisms and fungi account for a small percentage. (*1, p 354*)

13.9 (B) The microbiology of native valve endocarditis in intravenous drug users differs from that of other patients. *S. aureus* accounts for 60% or more of all cases and for 80% to 90% of cases in which the tricuspid valve is infected. (*1, p 354*)

13.10 (C) Blood culture is the single most important procedure for diagnosis of infective endocarditis. The incidence of positive cultures depends primarily on the etiologic agent and whether antibiotics have been administered. (*1, p 354*)

13.11 (D) The six identified human herpes viruses include herpes simplex virus (HSV) type 1, HSV type 2, varicella zoster virus (type 3), Epstein-Barr (EB) infectious mononucleosis virus (type 4), and cytomegalovirus (CMV) (type 5). A sixth agent (HHV-6) has been identified as the cause of roseola (exanthema subitum). Toxoplasmosis is an obligate intracellular protozoan found worldwide in humans and in many species of animals and birds. (*1, p 1353*)

13.12 (C) Mumps is associated with painful, swollen salivary glands, usually the parotids. Poliomyelitis is associated with muscle weakness, headache, stiff neck, fever, nausea and vomiting, and sore throat. Rubella is associated with no prodrome in children (mild in adults) and mild symptoms (fever, malaise, coryza) coinciding with eruption. (*1, p 1241*)

13.13 (D) RSV causes annual outbreaks of pneumonia, bronchiolitis, and tracheobronchitis. Reinfection is common and manifests itself typically as a mild URI and tracheobronchitis in older children or adults. In infants, diagnosis of lower respiratory tract disease may often be made on the basis of clinical and epidemiologic findings. Rapid diagnosis may be made by viral antigen identification of nasal washings using an ELISA or immunofluorescent assay. (*1*, *p 1255*)

13.14 (A) *R. rickettsii* is transmitted to humans by the bite of ticks, including the wood tick *D. andersoni* in the western United States and the dog tick *D. variabilis* in the eastern United States. *R. akari* is a parasite of mice that is transmitted by mites. (*1*, *p 1259*)

13.15 (A) Erysipelas is described as edematous, spreading, circumscribed, hot, and erythematous. Vesicle or bulla formation may or may not occur. The face is frequently involved. There may be pain, chills, and/or fever, and systemic toxicity may be striking. (*1*, *p 153*)

13.16 (A) Gas gangrene, or clostridial myonecrosis, is caused by entry of one of several clostridia (*C. perfringens, Clostridium ramosum, Clostridium bifermentans, Clostridium histolyticum, Clostridium novji,* etc.) into devitalized tissues. (*1*, *p 1275*)

13.17 (B) The presence of fever and bloody diarrhea (dysentery) indicates colonic tissue damage caused by invasion (shigellosis, salmonellosis, campylobacter or yersinia infection, amebiasis) or a toxin (*Clostridium difficile, Escherichia coli*). (*1*, *p 542*)

13.18 (A) For uncomplicated gonococcal urethritis or cervicitis, ceftriaxone 125 mg IM is the treatment of choice. Since coexistent chlamydial infection is common, erythromycin 500 mg four times daily orally, or doxycycline 100 mg twice daily orally for 7 days, is also used. (*1*, *p 1291*)

13.19 (C)   Chancroid is a sexually transmitted disease caused by the short gram-negative bacillus *H. ducreyi.* Granuloma inguinale is a chronic, relapsing granulomatous anogenital infection due to *C. granulomatis. (1, p 1292)*

13.20 (A)   Mycobacterium tuberculosis is not considered atypical. The following are considered atypical: *M. marinum* infection ("swimming pool granuloma") presents as a nodular skin lesion following exposure to nonchlorinated water. *M. kansasii* can produce clinical disease that resembles tuberculosis but progresses more slowly. *M. fortuitum* may cause skin and soft tissue infections such as abscesses, septic arthritis, and osteomyelitis. *(1, p 1296)*

13.21 (D)   Lymph node enlargement, softening, and suppuration with draining sinuses is a common finding with *C. trachomatis. (1, p 1301)*

13.22 (C)   Penicillin, as benzathine penicillin G or aqueous procaine penicillin G, is the drug of choice for all forms of syphilis and other spirochetal infections. *(1, p 1308)*

13.23 (D)   Generalized maculopapular skin rash is associated with secondary syphilis. *(1, p 1309)*

13.24 (D)   Meningitis, hepatitis, osteitis, and iritis are characteristic of secondary syphilis. *(1, p 1310)*

13.25 (A)   *T. brucei rhodesiense* causes sleeping sickness. Leptospirosis is an acute and often severe infection that frequently affects the liver or other organs and is caused by serovars of *L. interrogans. (1, p 1318)*

13.26 (D)   Some patients have an acute onset of severe diarrhea as early as 8 days (commonly 2 to 4 wk) after infection, requiring hospitalization. *(1, pp 1327–1330)*

13.27 (D)   Most infections are asymptomatic. Upper abdominal discomfort, cramps, distention, excessive flatus, and cysts and occasionally trophozoites in the stool characterize giardiasis. *(1, p 1337)*

13.28 (B) Humans are frequently infected by beef, pork, fish, dwarf, rodent, and dog tapeworms. (*1, p 1362*)

13.29 (A) Pinworm infection is found most often in young children. (*1, p 1374*)

13.30 (C) Hookworms infect 25% of the world's population. (*1, p 1377*)

Reference

1. Tierney LM, McPhee SJ, Papadakis MA: *Current Medical Diagnosis & Treatment,* 37/e, Stamford, CT, Appleton & Lange, 1998.

14

Liver Disease

Roberto Canales, MS, PA-C

DIRECTIONS (Questions 14.1–14.20): Each of the numbered items or incomplete statements in this chapter is followed by answers or completions of the statement. Select the **one** lettered answer or completion that is **best** in each case.

14.1 Physical exam findings of vascular spiders, palmar erythema, ascites, gynecomastia, sparse body hair, and asterixis are most likely associated with which of the following?
   A. Hereditary cholestatic syndromes
   B. Intrahepatic cholestasis
   C. Hepatocellular disease
   D. Biliary obstruction

14.2 Which of the following is **TRUE** regarding laboratory studies for the evaluation of liver disease?
   A. Alanine aminotransferase (ALT) is more specific for liver injury than aspartate aminotransferase (AST).
   B. Decreased alkaline phosphatase levels suggest cholestasis or infiltrative liver disease.
   C. Elevated serum AST and ALT levels may result from hepatocellular necrosis or inflammation.
   D. Prothrombin time is not a useful marker for liver disease severity.

14.3 Which viral hepatitis agent was formerly termed enterically transmitted non-A, non-B hepatitis, and is responsible for waterborne hepatitis outbreaks in India, Burma, Afghanistan, Algeria, and Mexico?
A. Hepatitis A
B. Hepatitis B
C. Hepatitis E
D. Delta agent (hepatitis D)

14.4 Which viral hepatitis agent is a defective RNA virus that causes hepatitis only in association with hepatitis B infection?
A. Hepatitis A
B. Hepatitis B
C. Hepatitis C
D. Delta agent (hepatitis D)

14.5 Which viral hepatitis agent is a single-stranded RNA virus with properties similar to those of flavivirus?
A. Hepatitis A
B. Hepatitis B
C. Hepatitis C
D. Delta agent (hepatitis D)

14.6 Which viral hepatitis is transmitted by the fecal-oral route and is enhanced by crowding and/or poor sanitation?
A. Hepatitis A
B. Hepatitis B
C. Hepatitis C
D. Delta agent (hepatitis D)

14.7 Which viral hepatitis agent is usually transmitted by inoculation of infected blood or blood products?
A. Hepatitis A
B. Hepatitis B
C. Hepatitis G
D. Hepatitis E

14.8 Which of the following conditions best describes hepatitis that takes a rapidly progressive course, terminating in death in less than 10 days to 8 wk, with up to 50% of cases being due to hepatitis B?

A. Cholestatic hepatitis
B. Hepatic carcinoma
C. Fulminant hepatitis
D. Chronic active hepatitis

14.9 Which of the following statements best describes alcoholic hepatitis?
A. It is often a nonreversible disease.
B. It is an uncommon precursor to cirrhosis.
C. Alcoholic hepatitis and cirrhosis do not develop in all chronic heavy drinkers.
D. Men appear to be more susceptible than women.

14.10 Which of the following is least likely to be a complication of cirrhosis?
A. Ascites
B. Renal insufficiency
C. Anemia
D. Hemorrhagic tendency

14.11 Which of the following statements is most consistent with Wilson's disease?
A. It is characterized by increased accumulation of iron hemosiderin in the liver, pancreas, heart, adrenals, testes, pituitary, and kidneys.
B. This uncommon disorder is due to occlusion of the hepatic veins from a variety of causes, such as polycythemia vera or other myeloproliferative diseases.
C. It is a chronic disease of the liver manifested by cholestasis.
D. It is a rare autosomal recessive disorder that usually occurs between the first and third decades and is characterized by excessive deposition of copper in the liver and brain.

14.12 Hepatocellular carcinomas are associated with which of the following?
A. Cirrhosis
B. Hepatitis B or C
C. Hemochromatosis
D. All of the above

14.13 Which of the following best describes epigastric abdominal pain, generally abrupt in onset, that is steady and severe, is often made worse by walking or lying supine, and is made better by sitting or leaning forward?
A. Acute cholecystitis
B. Acute pancreatitis
C. Chronic cholecystitis
D. Chronic pancreatitis

14.14 Which of the following conditions is most consistent with palmar erythema, spider angiomas, and testicular atrophy?
A. Portal hypertension
B. Gastrointestinal bleeding
C. Chronic liver disease
D. Acute hepatitis

14.15 What clinical condition best describes hepatitis that is generally a disease of young women, is insidious in onset, and may result in a positive test for HLA-B8, ANA, and elevated serum gamma globulin levels?
A. α_1 antitrypsin
B. Chronic cholecystitis
C. Autoimmune hepatitis
D. Portal hypertension

14.16 Which of the following clinical conditions is an autosomal recessive disorder that results in lung and liver disease in children and young adults?
A. α_1 antitrypsin
B. Chronic cholecystitis
C. Autoimmune hepatitis
D. Portal hypertension

14.17 Which of the following clinical conditions may present with ascites, splenomegaly, and vascular collaterals?
A. α_1 antitrypsin
B. Chronic cholecystitis
C. Autoimmune hepatitis
D. Portal hypertension

14.18 Which clinical condition best describes recurrent discrete episodes of epigastric or right upper quadrant pain that is described as steady and sudden in onset, persists for up to 3 h, and radiates to the shoulder or neck?
A. Chronic pancreatitis
B. Chronic cholecystitis
C. Acute appendicitis
D. Small bowel obstruction

14.19. Which of the following statements is **TRUE** regarding liver biopsy?
A. It is of little use.
B. Patterns of necrosis and scarring in the liver parenchyma have little prognostic importance.
C. Drug-induced granulomas and fatty infiltration can be confirmed by liver biopsy.
D. Bile stasis is a frequent finding in pure cholestasis due to estrogen therapy.

14.20. Which of the following statements is **FALSE** regarding the prognosis of alcoholic cirrhosis?
A. Diuretics and paracentesis are used to treat edema and ascites.
B. Antibiotics are required for spontaneous bacterial peritonitis.
C. Low-protein diets, lactulose, or neomycin are the usual treatments for hepatic encephalopathy.
D. There is little available management for variceal hemorrhage and bleeding from congestive gastropathy.

Liver Disease

Answers and Discussion

14.1 (C) Hereditary cholestatic syndromes or intrahepatic cholestasis are associated with pruritus, light-colored stools, and occasionally malaise. The patient may also be asymptomatic. With biliary obstruction, there may be colicky right upper quadrant pain, weight loss (carcinoma), jaundice, dark urine, and light-colored stools. (*1, p 636*)

14.2 (C) ALT is more specific for the liver than AST. Elevated alkaline phosphatase levels suggest cholestasis or infiltrative liver disease (e.g., tumor, abscess, granulomas). Prothrombin time is prolonged if damage is severe. (*1, p 631*)

14.3 (C) Hepatitis E is self-limited (no carrier state). (*1, p 633*)

14.4 (D) Hepatitis D is a defective RNA virus that causes hepatitis only in association with hepatitis B infection. (*1, p 633*)

14.5 (C) (*1, p 633*)

14.6 (A) (*1, p 631*)

14.7 (B) Hepatitis B is usually transmitted by inoculation of infected blood or blood products or by sexual contact and is present in saliva, semen, and vaginal secretions. (*1, p 631*)

14.8 (C) Fulminant hepatic failure is characterized by the development of hepatic encephalopathy within 8 wk after the onset of acute liver disease. It carries a poor prognosis, and up to 50% of cases are due to hepatitis B. (*1, p 635*)

14.9 (C) While alcoholic hepatitis is often a reversible disease, it is the most common precursor of cirrhosis in the United States, and cirrhosis ranks among the most common causes of death of adults in this country. Women appear to be more susceptible than men, in part because of lower gastric mucosal alcohol dehydrogenase levels. (*1, p 638*)

14.10 (B) Ascites and edema occur due to sodium retention, hypoproteinemia, and portal hypertension. There is an association with iron-deficiency anemia. A bleeding tendency due to hypoprothrombinemia may be treated with vitamin K preparations. Hepatic encephalopathy is a state of disordered central nervous system function resulting from failure of the liver to detoxify noxious agents of gut origin because of hepatocellular dysfunction and portosystemic shunting. (*1, p 624*)

14.11 (D) Hemochromatosis is characterized by increased accumulation of iron hemosiderin in the liver, pancreas, heart, adrenals, testes, pituitary, and kidneys. Primary biliary cirrhosis is a chronic disease of the liver manifested by cholestasis. Hepatic vein obstruction is an uncommon disorder that is due to occlusion of the hepatic veins from a variety of causes. (*1, p 647*)

14.12 (D) Hepatocellular carcinomas are associated with cirrhosis in general and with hepatitis B or C in particular. In Africa and Asia, hepatitis B is of major etiologic significance, whereas, in the Western countries and Japan, hepatitis C and alcoholic cirrhosis are the most common causes. Other associations include hemochromatosis. (*1, p 650*)

14.13 (B) An attack of acute cholecystitis is often precipitated by a large or fatty meal. It is characterized by the relatively sudden appearance of severe, minimally fluctuating pain that is localized to the epigastrum or right hypochondrium. Chronic cholecystitis may be associated with discrete bouts of right hypochondriac and epigastric pain that is either steady or intermittent. Persistent or recurrent episodes of epigastric and left upper quadrant pain with referral to the upper left lumbar region are typical for chronic pancreatitis. (*1, p 659*)

14.14 (C) Stigmata of chronic liver disease include palmar erythema, spider angiomas, and testicular atrophy. (*1, p 636*)

14.15 (C) Autoimmune hepatitis is generally a disease of young women who test positive for HLA-B8 and DR3. Classic type I patients will also test positive for ANA and elevated serum gamma globulin levels. (*1, p 636*)

14.16 (A) (*2, p 147*)

14.17 (D) Noncirrhotic portal hypertension may cause splenomegaly or upper gastrointestinal bleeding due to esophageal or gastric varices. Cirrhotic portal hypertension may cause ascites in addition to the symptoms previously mentioned. (*1, p 649*)

14.18 (B) The symptoms associated with chronic cholecystitis may be vaguely or indirectly related to gallbladder dysfunction. The pain may be epigastric (either steady or intermittent), may last several hours, and/or may be referred to the interscapular area or shoulder. (*1, p 655*)

14.19 (C) Liver biopsy may be helpful; patterns of necrosis and scarring in the liver parenchyma have prognostic importance; and bile stasis may be the only finding in pure cholestasis due to estrogen therapy. (*1, p 628*)

14.20 (D) Variceal hemorrhage and bleeding from congestive gastropathy are managed with sclerotherapy or portal-caval shunting. (*1, p 638*)

References

1. Tierney LM, McPhee SJ, Papadakis MA: *Current Medical Diagnosis & Treatment,* 37/e, Stamford, CT, Appleton & Lange, 1998.

2. Kelley NW: *Essentials of Internal Medicine.* Philadelphia, Lippincott, 1994.

15

Gastroenterology

J. Dennis Blessing, PhD, PA-C

DIRECTIONS (Questions 15.1–15.30): Each of the numbered items or incomplete statements in this chapter is followed by answers or completions of the statement. Select the **one** lettered answer or completion that is **best** in each case.

15.1 Which of the following is **NOT** a common cause of constipation?
   A. Narcotics
   B. Diuretics
   C. Antacids
   D. High-fiber diet
   E. Calcium channel blockers

15.2 In managing the adult patient with mild, self-limited diarrhea, recommendations for oral intake should include which of the following?
   A. High-fiber foods
   B. Tea
   C. Alcohol
   D. Milk
   E. All of the above

15.3 The most common cause of upper gastrointestinal bleeding is
   A. Peptic ulcer disease
   B. Portal hypertension
   C. Mallory-Weiss tears
   D. Gastric neoplasms
   E. Erosive esophagitis

15.4 Which of the following is **NOT** a sign or symptom of gastroesophageal reflux disease?
   A. Heartburn
   B. Heartburn made worse by standing
   C. Heartburn made worse by meals
   D. Heartburn relieved by antacids
   E. Heartburn 30 to 60 min after eating

15.5 Treatment of gastroesophageal reflux disease can include
   A. Avoidance of irritating foods
   B. Antacids
   C. H_2 receptor antagonists
   D. Proton pump inhibitors
   E. All of the above

15.6 Which is true of esophageal varices?
   A. They are rarely found in patients with liver cirrhosis.
   B. Diagnosis is established by barium swallow.
   C. They develop secondary to portal hypertension.
   D. They are rarely a source of upper GI bleeding.
   E. Levels of mortality from variceal hemorrhage are low.

15.7 Patients with gastric peptic ulcers should have endoscopic evaluation 12 wk after diagnosis and treatment because
   A. Gastric ulcers heal much more slowly than duodenal ulcers.
   B. Gastric ulcers may not cause any symptoms.
   C. Gastric ulcers always have bacterial etiologies.
   D. Gastric ulcers are malignant at a rate of 3% to 5%.
   E. Gastric ulcers never perforate.

15.8 A patient known to have a peptic ulcer develops severe abdominal pain, a board-like abdomen, hypoactive bowel sounds, and leucocytosis. The most likely diagnosis is
  A. Appendicitis
  B. Bleeding ulcer
  C. Ulcer perforation
  D. Secondary ulceration
  E. Gastritis

15.9 Zollinger-Ellison syndrome is characterized by
  A. Constipation
  B. Gastric acid hyposecretion
  C. Low fasting gastrin levels
  D. Low incidence of heartburn
  E. Peptic ulcers

15.10 The most common cause of intestinal obstruction is
  A. Surgical adhesions
  B. Bile ileus
  C. Intestinal carcinoma
  D. Colon diverticulum
  E. External injury

15.11 Which of the following would **NOT** be part of the classical presentation of acute appendicitis?
  A. Early periumbilical discomfort
  B. Right lower quadrant abdominal pain
  C. Nausea and vomiting
  D. WBC count over 20,000
  E. Low-grade temperature

15.12 A 25-year-old woman presents with complaints of abdominal distention and bloating; intermittent crampy abdominal pain relieved by defecation; and more frequent and loose stools when she has pain. She has not had any weight loss. She has had diarrhea on some occasions and constipation at other times. Her physical and laboratory examinations are unremarkable. The most likely diagnosis is
  A. Ulcerative colitis
  B. Crohn's disease

C. Chronic appendicitis
D. Viral gastroenteritis
E. Irritable bowel syndrome

15.13 The most common organism identified in patients with severe antibiotic-associated colitis is
A. *Clostridium difficile*
B. *Yersinia enterocolitica*
C. *Entamoeba histolytica*
D. Chlamydia
E. *Escherichia coli*

15.14 What is the difference between ulcerative colitis and Crohn's disease?
A. Ulcerative colitis involves only the rectum.
B. Crohn's disease may involve any part of the GI tract.
C. Crohn's disease is a small intestine disease.
D. Ulcerative colitis involves only the distal colon.
E. There is no difference between the two.

15.15 Which is true concerning the treatment of ulcerative colitis?
A. Without therapy, 75% of patients will relapse.
B. Treatment does not reduce risk of colon cancer.
C. Surgery is required for 25% of patients.
D. Treatment includes a high-fiber diet with restriction of gas-producing foods.
E. All of the above

15.16 Which is true of nonclinical colon diverticular disease?
A. The treatment of choice is colectomy.
B. Over two-thirds of people with diverticula require no treatment.
C. Acute disease requires surgery.
D. A low-fiber diet prevents acute episodes.
E. Drug prophylaxis is always indicated.

15.17 Which type of hepatitis has an increased incidence in chronic carriers?
   A. Hepatitis A
   B. Hepatitis B
   C. Hepatitis C
   D. Hepatitis D
   E. Hepatitis E

15.18 Treatment of mild cases of viral hepatitis includes all of the following **EXCEPT**
   A. Bed rest and reduction of activity
   B. Maintenance of hydration and nutrition
   C. Avoidance of hepatotoxins
   D. Broad-spectrum antibiotics
   E. Avoidance of intimate contact during viral shedding

15.19 When identified as the cause of an enteric infection, which organism requires antibiotic treatment?
   A. Salmonella
   B. Shigella
   C. E. coli
   D. Isospora belli
   E. Vibrio species

15.20 Which bacterium is a primary causative factor in peptic ulcer disease?
   A. E. coli
   B. Streptococcus equisimilis
   C. Staphylococcus aureus
   D. Helicobacter pylori

15.21 Which statement is true concerning diet and the occurrence of colorectal cancer?
   A. High-fiber diets increase risk.
   B. Animal fat is not a risk factor.
   C. Alcohol consumption increases risk.
   D. Fruits and vegetables do not affect risk.
   E. Red meat decreases risk.

15.22 The recommended screening procedure for individuals at high risk for developing colon cancer is
  A. Digital rectal examination
  B. Fecal occult blood test
  C. Barium enema
  D. Air-contrast barium enema
  E. Flexible colonoscopy

15.23 A patient presents with right upper quadrant pain that is described as sharp, but subsiding over 1 h. She has had several occurrences, usually after eating fatty foods. You suspect gallbladder disease. Which diagnostic study would you recommend first to confirm your diagnosis?
  A. Ultrasound of the gallbladder
  B. Oral cholecystography
  C. Percutaneous cholecystography
  D. Retrograde endoscopic cholangiography
  E. Exploratory surgery

15.24 A patient known to have gallstones presents with sharp right upper quadrant pain that started after the evening meal and lasted all night. He has had nausea, but has not vomited. Physical exam reveals low-grade fever, RUQ pain with positive Murphy sign, equivocal rebound tenderness, WBCs of 14,000, and elevated bilirubin. The most likely diagnosis is
  A. Acute hepatitis
  B. Acute pancreatitis
  C. Common duct obstruction
  D. Bacterial cholecystitis
  E. Acute pancreatitis

15.25 Which of the following is a complication of liver cirrhosis?
  A. Ascites
  B. Portal hypertension
  C. Esophageal varices
  D. Hepatic encephalopathy
  E. All of the above

15.26 Which of the following is **NOT** a component of the treatment of a patient with mild to moderate acute pancreatitis?
A. Hospitalization
B. Hydration and fluid replacement
C. Nothing by mouth (NPO)
D. High doses of broad-spectrum antibiotics
E. Nasogastric tube placement

15.27 Which historical clue would point to a diagnosis of duodenal peptic ulcer disease rather than gastric ulcer?
A. Pain made worse by eating
B. Pain on an empty stomach
C. No relief with antacids
D. Right lower quadrant pain
E. Presence of diarrhea

15.28 It is recommended that antibiotic therapy for the eradication of *H. pylori* in peptic ulcer disease include
A. Fiber supplements
B. Bismuth subsalicylate
C. Vitamin supplements
D. Milk of magnesia
E. Simethicone

15.29 Treatment for irritable bowel syndrome includes
A. Patient education
B. High-fiber diet
C. Behavior modification
D. Avoidance of irritating foods
E. All of the above

15.30 Which of the following is **NOT** a sign or symptom of ulcerative colitis?
A. Lower abdominal cramps/discomfort
B. Negative stool cultures
C. Constipation
D. Defecation urgency
E. All of the above

Gastroenterology

Answers and Discussion

15.1 (D) A careful review of diet generally shows that most constipated patients do not consume adequate amounts of fiber and fluids. (*1, pp 543–545*)

15.2 (B) Patients can rest the bowel by avoiding high-fiber foods, caffeine, alcohol, and milk. (*1, pp 546–549*)

15.3 (A) Peptic ulcer disease accounts for half of upper gastrointestinal bleeding. The acute mortality rate is 6% to 10%. (*1, pp 552–555*)

15.4 (B) Patients with gastroesophageal reflux disease should avoid lying down within 3 h of eating. (*1, pp 546–568*)

15.5 (E) Antacids, H_2 receptor antagonists, and avoidance of irritating foods may be used to treat gastroesophageal reflux disease. Proton pump inhibitors are used with erosive esophagitis. (*1, pp 564–568*)

15.6 (C) Esophageal varices develop secondary to portal hypertension. Diagnosis is established by upper endoscopy. (*1, pp 571–575*)

15.7 (D) Gastric ulcer biopsies should be performed 12 wk after the start of therapy, since nonhealing ulcers may be malignant. (*1, pp 583–589*)

15.8 (C) Perforations develop in 5% of peptic ulcer patients. (*1, pp 589–591*)

15.9 (E) Peptic ulcer disease may be severe in patients with Zollinger-Ellison syndrome. (*1, pp 592–593*)

15.10 (A) Postoperative adhesions and external hernia are the most common causes of acute organic small intestinal obstruction. (*1, pp 602–603*)

15.11 (D) A WBC count of 10,000 to 20,000 with increases in neutrophils is usually seen in acute appendicitis. (*1, pp 608–609*)

15.12 (E) The symptoms of irritable bowel disease are seen in almost 20% of the adult population. (*1, pp 610–613*)

15.13 (A) *C. difficile* is found in the stools of 15% to 25% of patients with antibiotic-associated colitis. However, most cases of antibiotic-associated diarrhea are not caused by the bacterium. (*1, pp 613–619*)

15.14 (B) Ulcerative colitis almost always involves the colon only. Crohn's disease can involve any segment of the GI tract. (*1, pp 614–622*)

15.15 (E) The goal of treatment for ulcerative colitis is symptomatic relief and reduction of inflammation, since there is no specific therapy. (*1, pp 619–622*)

15.16 (B) Patients with uncomplicated diverticulosis have no symptoms and require no treatment. (*1, pp 623–626*)

15.17 (C) Hepatitis C has increased incidence in common carriers. (*2, pp 25–36*)

15.18 (D) Broad spectrum antibiotics are ineffective for mild cases of viral hepatitis. (*2, pp 25–36*)

15.19 (B) Trimethoprin sulfamethoxazole or ciprofloxacin is the treatment of choice for shigellosis. (*3, pp 45–52*)

15.20 (D)   *H. pylori* is associated with the majority of ulcers not induced by NSAIDs. (*4, pp 38–45*)

15.21 (C)   Alcohol consumption and diets high in red meat and animal fat increase the risk of colorectal cancer. (*5, pp 15–39*)

15.22 (E)   Flexible colonoscopy can detect adenomatous polyps, which can then be biopsied. (*5, pp 15–39*)

15.23 (A)   Ultrasonography of the gallbladder is sensitive and specific for detecting gallbladder disease. (*6, pp 446–449*)

15.24 (C)   Gallstone obstruction of the common bile duct produces the symptoms. (*6, pp 446–449*)

15.25 (E)   Ascites, portal hypertension, esophageal varices, and hepatic encephalopathy are all complications of cirrhosis. (*7, pp 449–457*)

15.26 (D)   Mild to moderate acute pancreatitis can be treated with hospitalization and a bed rest program. Broad-spectrum antibiotics are not effective. (*8, pp 506–509*)

15.27 (B)   Pain on an empty stomach points to a duodenal peptic ulcer rather than a gastric ulcer. (*9, pp 524–529*)

15.28 (B)   Bismuth subsalicylate is part of the first-line treatment regimen for *H. pylori*–associated peptic ulcer disease. (*4, pp 38–45*)

15.29 (E)   Most patients respond to dietary changes and patient education about irritable bowel syndrome. Drug therapy is reserved for severe symptoms. (*1, pp 610–613*)

15.30 (C)   Constipation is not indicative of ulcerative colitis; bloody diarrhea is the most common sign. (*1, pp 619–622*)

References

1. McQuaid KR: Alimentary tract. In Tierney LM Jr, McPhee SJ, Papadakis MA (eds): *Current Medical Diagnosis & Treatment,* 38/e, Stamford, CT, Appleton & Lange, 1999.

2. Konigsberg AJ: Keeping up with viral hepatitis. *Physician Assist* 16(7):25–36, 1992.

3. Lipsky S: The role of PAs in the surveillance and management of enteric infections. *Physician Assist* 18(2):45–52, 1994.

4. Fedotin MS: *Helicobacter pylori* and peptic ulcer disease. *Postgrad Med* 94(3):38–45, 1993.

5. Hansen C: Colorectal cancer, a preventable disease. *Physician Assist* 19(1):15–39, 1995.

6. Nahrwold DL: Cholelithiasis and cholecystitis. In: Rakel RE (ed): *Conn's Current Therapy,* Philadelphia, Saunders, 1998.

7. Reynolds TB: Cirrhosis. In: Rakel RE (ed): *Conn's Current Therapy,* Philadelphia, Saunders, 1998.

8. Bunch JM: Acute pancreatitis. In: Rakel RE (ed), *Conn's Current Therapy,* Philadelphia, Saunders, 1998.

9. Achord JL: Peptic ulcer disease. In: Rakel RE (ed): *Conn's Current Therapy,* Philadelphia, Saunders, 1998.

16

Dermatology

J. Dennis Blessing, PhD, PA-C

DIRECTIONS (Questions 16.1–16.20): Each of the numbered items or incomplete statements in this chapter is followed by answers or completions of the statement. Select the **one** lettered answer or completion that is **best** in each case.

16.1 The addition of topical antibiotics to the treatment of acne in combination with oral antibiotics
   A. Is not beneficial
   B. Decreases time to resolution
   C. Prevents development of resistant organisms
   D. Has a strong anti-inflammatory effect

16.2 A diagnostic clue to contact dermatitis caused by an irritant versus an allergic reaction is that contact dermatitis
   A. Is less erythemic
   B. Lacks wheals
   C. Is less pruritic
   D. Shows localized involvement
   E. Involves systemic reaction

16.3 The most common area for presentation of the lesions of atopic dermatitis in infants is the
A. Extremities
B. Cheeks
C. Trunk
D. Scalp

16.4 The most likely diagnosis for lesions that appear on the elbows and knees, described as almost circular, erythemic plaques with silver-white scales, is
A. Erythema multiforme
B. Psoriasis
C. Pityriasis rosea
D. Angioedema
E. Lymphangitis

16.5 The most likely diagnosis for a lesion on a 12-year-old described as a sharply marginated, erythematous plaque with a clear or clearing center is
A. Tinea pedis
B. Tinea versicolor
C. Tinea cruris
D. Tinea corporis
E. Tinea capitis

16.6 Which of the following is **NOT** true about impetigo?
A. It is caused by streptococcal and staphylococcal bacteria.
B. It appears as thick, honey-colored crusts.
C. It occurs primarily in children.
D. Any area of the skin may be affected.
E. It is noncontagious.

16.7 Postherpetic pain from herpes zoster may be relieved by which of the following as an adjunct to other therapy?
A. Tricyclic antidepressants
B. Antianxiety medications
C. Antibiotics
D. Diuretics
E. Varicella immunization

16.8 Common warts can be
   A. Excised
   B. Treated by electrodesiccation
   C. Treated by liquid nitrogen application
   D. Allowed to resolve spontaneously
   E. All of the above

16.9 Often, mild to moderate acne can be managed with
   A. Topical therapy alone
   B. Daily washing with hypoallergenic soap
   C. Oral steroids
   D. Dermabrasion

16.10 What is the most likely diagnosis for a lesion described as beginning as a small nodule whose center, as the lesion enlarges, becomes ulcerated and develops a pearly, rolled border?
   A. Basal cell carcinoma
   B. Squamous cell carcinoma
   C. Melanoma
   D. Malignant lentigo
   E. Acanthoma

16.11 The most common precancerous lesions of the skin are
   A. Freckles
   B. Moles
   C. Actinic keratoses
   D. Scars
   E. Keratotic horns

16.12 The antibiotic of choice for the treatment of a furuncle (boil) is
   A. Doxycycline
   B. Erythromycin
   C. Sulfisoxazole
   D. Dicloxacillin
   E. Penicillin VK

16.13 Which antibiotic ointment is highly effective against the organisms that cause impetigo?
   A. Benzoyl peroxide
   B. Tretinoin
   C. Erythromycin
   D. Mupirocin
   E. Metrogel

16.14 A diffuse, poorly demarcated inflammation of the subcutaneous tissue with erythema, warmth, and tenderness best describes
   A. Furunculosis
   B. Lymphangitis
   C. Cellulitis
   D. Impetigo
   E. Folliculitis

16.15 The major risk factor for the development of skin cancer is
   A. Smog and air pollution exposure
   B. Repeated exposure to ultraviolet (sun) light
   C. Smoking more than three packs of cigarettes per day
   D. Lack of exposure to sunlight
   E. Repeated use of steroid-containing ointments

16.16 Which of the following drugs is most likely to produce photosensitivity?
   A. Aspirin
   B. Tetracycline
   C. Penicillin
   D. Antihistamines

16.17 The presence of a herald patch is diagnostic of
   A. Erythema multiforme
   B. Tinea versicolor
   C. Erythema migrans
   D. Measles
   E. Pityriasis rosea

16.18 Guttate psoriasis is associated with what type of infection?
   A. Streptococcal
   B. Staphylococcal
   C. Fungal
   D. Viral
   E. Coliform

16.19 Which of the following statements is **NOT** true about Kaposi's sarcoma in the HIV-positive individual?
   A. It can affect any organ.
   B. It presents in a variety of forms, shapes, and colors.
   C. It is typically nonpruritic and painless.
   D. It occurs only with low T4 counts.
   E. Patients usually relapse quickly after therapy.

16.20 Acute urticaria usually
   A. Takes 7 to 10 days to resolve
   B. Is intensely pruritic
   C. Has vesicular lesions
   D. Responds to oral steroids
   E. Occurs with angioedema

Dermatology

Answers and Discussion

ŗ

16.1 (A) Combining topical and oral antibiotics in the treatment of acne is of no benefit. Use of both oral and topical antibiotics and preparations offers no benefit and may increase the likelihood of developing antibiotic-resistant bacteria. (*1, p 35*)

16.2 (D) In addition to localized involvement, irritant dermatitis often appears red and scaly, whereas allergic dermatitis typically presents with weeping and crusting. Impetigo is the diagnosis most often confused with contact dermatitis. (*2, p 5*)

16.3 (B) In infants, lesions of atopic dermatitis commonly present on the cheeks. Atopic dermatitis must be distinguished from seborrheic dermatitis, which also involves the face among infants. (*2, p 7*)

16.4 (B) The combination of erythemic plaques with silver-white scales on the elbows and knees and scaliness of the scalp is diagnostic for psoriasis. (*2, p 8*)

16.5 (D) Fungal studies will distinguish tinea corporis from other skin lesions with annular shapes. (*2, p 11*)

16.6 (E) Impetigo, while occurring most often in children, is highly contagious; adults can be infected. (*2, p 14*)

236

16.7 (A) Tricyclic antidepressants can be used for postzoster neuralgia. (*2, p 17*)

16.8 (E) Warts can be treated in a variety of ways. A key treatment goal is to avoid scarring. Fifty percent of warts spontaneously resolve. (*2, p 19*)

16.9 (A) Early inflammatory lesions respond to topical therapies with or without antibiotics. (*1, pp 33–35*)

16.10 (A) Squamous cell carcinoma lesions are not as easy to distinguish as basal cell carcinoma lesions. (*3, pp 101–111*)

16.11 (C) Approximately 0.1% of actinic keratoses per year become squamous cell carcinomas. (*4, pp 115–126*)

16.12 (D) Dicloxacillin is the antibiotic treatment of choice for furuncles. Cephalin is an alternative. (*5, pp 43–52*)

16.13 (D) Topical mupirocin is highly effective. If the affected area is very large, or if there is toxicity or fever, a systemic antibiotic is indicated. (*5, pp 43–52*)

16.14 (C) Cellulitis involves deeper tissues than other skin infections. (*5, pp 43–52*)

16.15 (B) Repeated exposure to ultraviolet radiation—usually from the sun, but also in tanning booths—is the major risk factor for developing skin cancer. (*6, pp 80–94*)

16.16 (B) In addition to tetracyclines, sulfonamides may produce photosensitivity. (*6, pp 80–94*)

16.17 (E) In pityriasis rosea, a herald patch usually precedes the eruption by 1 to 2 wk. (*7, p 98*)

16.18 (A) Guttate (eruptive) psoriasis is associated with streptococcal infection. (*7, p 92*)

16.19 (D) Kaposi's sarcoma can occur with normal T4 counts. (*8, pp 133–134*)

16.20 (B) Acute urticaria incidents usually resolve in 1 to 2 wk. Itching is usually very intense, but in rare cases may be absent. (*9, pp 75–85*)

References

1. Thiboutot DM: Acne. In Arndt KA, et al (eds): *Primary Care Dermatology*, Philadelphia, Saunders, 1997.

2. Zarbock SR (ed): *Common Dermatologic Disorders in Primary Care*, Alexandria, VA, American Academy of Physician Assistants, 1995.

3. Hacker SM, Browder JF, Ramos-Caro FA: Basal cell carcinoma. *Postgrad Med* 93(8):101–111, 1993.

4. Hacker SM, Flowers FP: Squamous cell carcinoma of the skin. *Postgrad Med* 93(8):115–126, 1993.

5. Hacker SM: Common infections of the skin. *Postgrad Med* 96(2):43–52, 1994.

6. Korn K: Suntan and ultraviolet light exposure–related issues. *Physician Assist* 19(5):80–94, 1995.

7. Forbes CD, Jackson WF: *Color Atlas and Text of Clinical Medicine*, St. Louis, Mosby-Year Book, 1993.

8. Roquemore SW, Wegmann A, Ayachi S: Dermatologic manifestations. In Muma RD et al: *HIV Manual for Health Care Professionals*, Norwalk, CT, Appleton & Lange, 1994.

9. Pariser RJ: Allergic and reactive dermatoses. *Postgrad Med* 89(8):75–85, 1991.

17

Geriatrics

Karen S. Stephenson, MS, PA-C

DIRECTIONS (Questions 17.1–17.30): Each of the numbered items or incomplete statements in this chapter is followed by answers or completions of the statement. Select the **one** lettered answer or completion that is **best** in each case.

17.1 Which of the following is **NOT** one of the cardiovascular changes expected during maximal exercise in the elderly?
   A. Decrease in heart rate
   B. Decrease in stroke volume
   C. Increase in end-diastolic volume
   D. Cardiac hypertrophy

17.2 All of the following describe differences between the depressed elderly and younger adults **EXCEPT**
   A. Loss of self-esteem
   B. Inability to concentrate
   C. Psychological instead of somatic symptoms
   D. Impaired memory and cognition

17.3 Even though insomnia is a common sign of depression in the elderly, all of the following changes in sleep patterns are normal for the elderly **EXCEPT**

A. Shorter time for the onset of sleep
B. Earlier bedtime
C. Decrease in deeper stages of sleep
D. Increased periods of wakefulness

17.4 If, after investigation, the sleep patterns are abnormal and a diagnosis of depression is established, what considerations about the effects of antidepressive drugs are important? Choose the answer **NOT** specific to the elderly.
A. Dosage of the drug
B. Half-life of the drug
C. Level of sedation
D. Sympathetic action

17.5 All of the following are expected changes in the kidney among the elderly **EXCEPT**
A. Loss of tissue from the renal cortex
B. Decrease in renal blood flow
C. Decrease in glomerular flow rate
D. Rise in serum creatinine

17.6 Using the formula for creatinine clearance rate, what is the rate for a 70-year-old man who weighs 70 kg and has a creatinine of 1.1? The formula is $(140 - age) \times$ weight in kg $\div (72 \times$ serum creatinine). For women, multiply by 0.85.
A. 42
B. 52
C. 62
D. 72

17.7 Which of the following protects the elderly patient from urinary tract infections?
A. High vaginal pH
B. Prostatic secretions
C. Decline in renal function
D. Bladder prolapse

17.8 Which of the following characteristics does **NOT** contribute to eradication of bacteria from the urinary tract over a long period of time?
  A. Functional status
  B. Place of residence
  C. Underlying disease
  D. Use of antibiotics

17.9 Enlargement of the prostate can lead to all of the following symptoms **EXCEPT**
  A. Dribbling of urine
  B. Relaxed urinary meatus
  C. Urinary retention
  D. Nocturia

17.10 Which of the following organisms is associated with peptic ulcer disease and cancer of the stomach?
  A. *Helicobacter pylori*
  B. *Moraxella catarrhalis*
  C. Monilia
  D. Streptococcus

17.11 Nonsteroidals damage the gastric mucosa by what mechanism?
  A. Decreased production of saliva
  B. Decreased production of bile
  C. Decreased production of prostaglandins
  D. Decreased production of lipase

17.12 All of the following statements about acute cholecystitis in the elderly are true **EXCEPT**
  A. The condition is caused by obstruction of the cystic duct by stones.
  B. There may be no abdominal tenderness or peritoneal signs.
  C. *Staphylococcus aureus* is the most common causative organism.
  D. Many patients who appear ill already have gangrene or perforation.

17.13 All of the following statements about diverticular disease in the elderly are true **EXCEPT**
  A. It is associated with a drop in dietary fiber in the diets of Americans.
  B. Symptoms of inflammation include colicky pain and right lower quadrant pain.
  C. The symptoms of diverticulitis may mask advanced cancer of the colon.
  D. Most diverticula are asymptomatic.

17.14 All of the following statements about acute diverticulitis in the elderly are true **EXCEPT**
  A. Fever may be absent.
  B. No bleeding is present.
  C. There is little rise in white count.
  D. There is no pain or mass upon examination.

17.15 Most cancers of the colon occur in which region of the colon?
  A. Right
  B. Transverse
  C. Left
  D. Sigmoid

17.16 These left-sided cancers are more likely to present with all of the following **EXCEPT**
  A. Hematochezia
  B. Occult bleeding
  C. Change in size of stool
  D. Constipation or diarrhea

17.17 All of the following foods may make a stool guaiac positive **EXCEPT**
  A. Broccoli
  B. Cauliflower
  C. Bread
  D. Red meats

17.18 When prescribing digoxin for an elderly patient, which of the following concerns does **NOT** affect use of the drug?
A. Half-life of the drug
B. Renal clearance rates
C. Percentage of adipose tissue
D. Plasma-binding protein

17.19 All of the following statements about macrocytic anemia in the elderly are true **EXCEPT**
A. One form is pernicious anemia that results from low B_{12} levels.
B. Folate deficiencies usually result from loss of intrinsic factor.
C. Lack of B_{12} may cause peripheral neuropathy, ataxia, or upper motor neuron signs.
D. The patient may be demented.

17.20 Neutrophils perform which of the following functions?
A. Antibody production
B. Antigen processing
C. Bacteria phagocytosis
D. Cytokine production

17.21 Which of the following is considered the most reliable in detecting hypothyroidism in the elderly?
A. FT_4 index
B. TSH
C. T_3
D. T_4

17.22 Replacement of thyroid hormone in the elderly must be done slowly due to the potential to precipitate
A. Cardiac arrythmias
B. Myxedema
C. Renal failure
D. Dementia

17.23 Which of the following fasting blood sugar levels is used to help diagnose diabetes in the elderly?
A. 110 mg/dL
B. 120 mg/dL

C. 130 mg/dL
D. 140 mg/dL

17.24 All of the following characteristics are found in women with osteoporosis **EXCEPT**
A. Advanced age
B. Low calcium levels
C. Loss of estrogen
D. Physical activity

17.25 A 70-year-old woman presents to your clinic with a 2-day history of unilateral temporal headache. Which one of the following would you **NOT** expect to find?
A. Shoulder/hip girdle stiffness
B. Fever
C. Weight gain
D. Claudication

17.26 Which of the following findings is **LESS** likely to occur in osteoarthritis than rheumatoid arthritis (RA)?
A. It is most likely in the hips and knees.
B. Symptoms are worse in the morning.
C. Joints may be large but without inflammation.
D. There may be few white cells in the synovium.

17.27 Methotrexate is a commonly used second-line treatment for RA. Which of the following is a common deficiency that arises from this drug?
A. Calcium loss
B. Folic acid loss
C. Ascorbic acid loss
D. Vitamin B_6 loss

17.28 Exercise accomplishes all of the following for the elderly with osteoarthritis **EXCEPT**
A. Shortens muscles
B. Restores strength
C. Decreases pain
D. Decreases limitation

17.29 Stress incontinence (loss of urine with coughing or Valsalva maneuver) can be caused by which of the following mechanisms?
   A. Anatomic obstruction
   B. Acontractile bladder
   C. Psychological factors
   D. Weakness of the pelvic floor

17.30 Which of the following is **NOT** an appropriate treatment for stress incontinence?
   A. α-adrenergic agonists
   B. Bladder relaxants
   C. Estrogen
   D. Pelvic floor exercises

Geriatrics

Answers and Discussion

17.1 (B) The stroke volume becomes slightly increased so as to maintain cardiac output. Cardiomegaly may result from this. (*1, pp 257–258*)

17.2 (C) The elderly are more likely to present with somatic complaints than psychological ones. (*1, p 131*)

17.3 (A) In the elderly, the time from lying down until the onset of sleep is lengthened rather than shortened. All of the other changes are normal but may concern elderly persons, who may think something is now wrong with their sleep. (*1, p 122*)

17.4 (D) Antidepressants have anticholinergic properties that create problems such as urinary retention and acute angle glaucoma in the elderly. (*1, pp 138–139*)

17.5 (D) Even though creatinine clearance rate falls with age, the amount of creatinine produced decreases with a smaller muscle mass. Therefore, the serum creatinine would not rise even in an individual with a higher creatinine clearance rate. (*2, p 616*)

17.6 (C) If the patient were 30 years old with the same descriptions as in question 17.4, his creatinine clearance would be

97. If the patient were a woman, her value would be 53. (*1, pp 363, 371*)

17.7 (B) Loss of estrogen in females leads to high vaginal pH and bladder prolapse. Decline in renal function leads to loss of acidity of the urine, which also protects against bacteriuria. (*2, pp 626–627*)

17.8 (D) Use of antibiotics does not usually cure bacteriuria if the patient lives in a nursing home, is dependent on others for care, and has an underlying disease. People who live independently and function well have a much lower rate of bacteria in the urine. (*2, p 630*)

17.9 (B) Other symptoms of prostate enlargement may include dysuria, frequency, hesitancy, and decreased urinary stream. (*3, p 658*)

17.10 (A) *H. pylori* is more prominent in developing countries, but 50% of Americans at age 60 have the organism in their stomachs. (*4, p 658*)

17.11 (C) The decreased production of prostaglandins leads to an altered gastric mucosal barrier. NSAIDs also interfere with platelet aggregation. (*4, p 694*)

17.12 (C) *Escherichia coli* and klebsiella are the most common organisms causing acute cholecystitis in the elderly. Patients may appear disoriented and in shock during an episode but have no abdominal signs, fever, or leucocytosis. (*4, p 711*)

17.13 (B) Most diverticulosis occurs in the left colon. (*5, p 724*)

17.14 (B) Blood may be present in diverticulitis, but it is usually occult. (*5, p 724*)

17.15 (C) Sixty percent of carcinomas are in the left area of the colon. (*5, p 727*)

17.16 (D) The other symptoms are consistent with left colon lesions. (*5, p 728*)

17.17 (C) Other foods that can cause false positives include turnips, radishes, and parsnips. Iron supplements and ascorbic acids can do so also. (*5, p 729*)

17.18 (C) Digoxin is water soluble, and lean muscle mass decreases with age. Decreased amounts of plasma-binding protein and declining renal clearance rates, as well as loss of lean body mass, may prolong the half-life of digoxin to twice that in a young adult (70 vs. 36 h). (*6, p 221*)

17.19 (B) Macrocytic anemia usually results from lack of folate in the diet. (*7, p 743*)

17.20 (C) These white cells engulf antigens; T-lymphocytes identify antigens; B-lymphocytes produce antibodies; cytokines serve as messengers between white cells. White cells lose some of their function in old age. (*8, p 743*)

17.21 (B) An elevated TSH and a low T_4 confirm the diagnosis, but the TSH level is considered the more sensitive indicator. (*9, p 817*)

17.22 (A) Dosage can begin with as little as 0.025 mg of thyroxine. Restoring a normal TSH is the end point for the thyroid dose, but may take longer in the elderly because of the low dose initially. (*9, p 818*)

17.23 (D) This level is recommended because it will identify all those with an abnormal oral glucose tolerance test. Those with glucose between 115 and 140 mg/dL may also have abnormal GTT and may need to be evaluated. (*10, p 830*)

17.24 (D) Physical activity helps maintain bone structure rather than deplete it. (*11, p 899*)

17.25 (C) These symptoms are caused by polymyalgia rheumatica, of which giant cell arteritis is a part. Treatment must be provided in order to prevent blindness from the arteritis. The usual drug is prednisone. (*12, p 957*)

17.26 (B) Even though there may be overlap between osteoarthritis and RA concerning pain in the morning, the stiffness of osteoarthritis is usually shorter-lasting than that of rheumatoid arthritis and then recurs later in the day with use. (*13, p 967*)

17.27 (B) The depletion of folic acid may lead to macrocytic anemia and nausea. (*13, p 968*)

17.28 (A) Muscles tend to shorten as we age, and exercise helps to combat that and to maintain alignment of the joints, especially the weight-bearing ones. (*13, p 968*)

17.29 (D) Bladder outlet or urethral sphincter weakness can also lead to stress incontinence. Anatomic factors (prostate, cystocele) and acontractile bladder can cause overflow incontinence. Psychological factors such as depression, anger, and hostility can cause functional incontinence. (*14, p 1232*)

17.30 (B) Both α-adrenergic agonists and bladder relaxants carry with them significant side effects, especially in the elderly. Neither drug works without the addition of estrogen, which aids in the return of the vaginal flora and appropriate angle of the bladder neck. Behavioral techniques combined with the two medications seem to work the best. (*14, pp 1240–1242*)

References

1. Kane RL, Ouslander JG, Abrass IB: *Essentials of Clinical Geriatrics,* 3/e, New York, McGraw-Hill, 1994.

2. Tunkel AR, Kaye D: Urinary tract infections. In: Hazzard WR, Bierman EL, Blass JP (eds): *Principles of Geriatric Medicine and Gerontology,* 3/e, New York, McGraw-Hill, 1994.

3. Brendler CB: Disorders of the prostate. In: Hazzard WR, Bierman EL, Blass JP (eds): *Principles of Geriatric Medicine and Gerontology,* 3/e, New York, McGraw-Hill, 1994.

4. Kerr RM: Disorders of the stomach and duodenum. In: Hazzard WR, Bierman EL, Blass JP (eds): *Principles of Geriatric Medicine and Gerontology,* 3/e, New York, McGraw-Hill, 1994.

5. Cheskin LJ, Schuster MM: Colonic disorders. In: Hazzard WR, Bierman EL, Blass JP (eds): *Principles of Geriatric Medicine and Gerontology,* 3/e, New York, McGraw-Hill, 1994.

6. Swonger AK, Burbank PM: *Drug Therapy and the Elderly.* Boston, Jones & Bartlett, 1995.

7. Lipschitz DA: Anemia. In: Hazzard WR, Bierman EL, Blass JP (eds): *Principles of Geriatric Medicine and Gerontology,* 3/e, New York, McGraw-Hill, 1994.

8. Rothstein G: White cell disorders. In: Hazzard WR, Bierman EL, Blass JP (eds): *Principles of Geriatric Medicine and Gerontology,* 3/e, New York, McGraw-Hill, 1994.

9. Gregerman RI, Katz MS: Thyroid diseases. In: Hazzard WR, Bierman EL, Blass JP (eds): *Principles of Geriatric Medicine and Gerontology,* 3/e, New York, McGraw-Hill, 1994.

10. Goldberg AP, Coon PJ: Diabetes mellitus and glucose metabolism in the elderly. In: Hazzard WR, Bierman EL, Blass JP (eds): *Principles of Geriatric Medicine and Gerontology,* 3/e, New York, McGraw-Hill, 1994.

11. Chestnut CH III: Osteoporosis. In: Hazzard WR, Bierman EL, Blass JP (eds): *Principles of Geriatric Medicine and Gerontology,* 3/e, New York, McGraw-Hill, 1994.

12. Eisenberg GM: Polymyalgia rheumatica and giant cell arteritis. In: Hazzard WR, Bierman EL, Blass JP (eds): *Principles of Geriatric Medicine and Gerontology,* 3/e, New York, McGraw-Hill, 1994.

13. Calkins E, Reinhard JD, Vladutiu AO: Rheumatoid arthritis and the autoimmune rheumatoid disease in the older patient. In: Hazzard WR, Bierman EL, Blass JP (eds): *Principles of Geriatric Medicine and Gerontology,* 3/e, New York, McGraw-Hill, 1994.

14. Ouslander JG: Incontinence. In: Hazzard WR, Bierman EL, Blass JP (eds): *Principles of Geriatric Medicine and Gerontology,* 3/e, New York, McGraw-Hill, 1994.

18

Hematology and Oncology

Frances Coulson, MS, PA-C

DIRECTIONS (Questions 18.1–18.50): Each of the numbered items or incomplete statements in this chapter is followed by answers or completions of the statement. Select the **one** lettered answer or completion that is **best** in each case.

18.1 Which of the following symptoms would be expected with anemia?
A. Fatigue
B. Depression
C. Cervical lymphadenopathy
D. Night sweats

18.2 Iron-deficiency anemia
A. May be caused by NSAID use
B. May be caused by koilonychia
C. Is characterized by hyperchromia
D. Is characterized by an increased MCV

18.3 Which test is most the appropriate first step to determine the status of erythropoiesis after anemia has been found?
  A. Bone marrow aspiration
  B. Serum ferritin
  C. Guaiac
  D. Reticulocyte count

18.4 Paresthesias, disturbances of proprioception, progressive dementia, and psychosis should alert the clinician to the possibility of
  A. Low iron stores
  B. Vitamin B_{12} deficiency
  C. Side effects of ferrous sulfate
  D. Internal bleeding

18.5 A 62-year-old African American woman presents with anorexia, glossitis, irritability, and general malaise. Labs reveal macrocytic anemia and neutrophil hypersegmentation with a reticulocyte count of less than 2%. Of the following, which is most likely?
  A. Iron-deficiency anemia
  B. Sickle cell anemia
  C. Pernicious anemia
  D. β thalassemia major

18.6 A 17-year-old African American girl reports to the emergency department with severe bone and joint pain. CBC shows moderately severe anemia and elevated leukocyte and platelet counts. What two tests would be used to confirm your suspicion of HbSS?
  A. Reticulocyte count and manual differential
  B. Peripheral blood smear and hemoglobin electrophoresis
  C. Joint aspiration and evaluation
  D. Liver biopsy

18.7 A patient with sickle cell trait might be expected to suffer intermittently from which of the following symptoms?
  A. Painless hematuria
  B. Bone pain
  C. Abdominal pain
  D. Jaundice

18.8 The thalassemia anemias are characterized by which of the following?
  A. They involve altered synthesis of the globin chains.
  B. They are most commonly found in the Nordic population.
  C. They are divided into β and δ thalassemia types.
  D. They always result in a shortened life span.

18.9 The Philadelphia chromosome is a classic feature of which of the following?
  A. Acute lymphocytic leukemia (ALL)
  B. Acute myelocytic leukemia (AML)
  C. Chronic lymphocytic leukemia (CLL)
  D. Chronic myelocytic leukemia (CML)

18.10 Which of the following is **TRUE** regarding the leukemias?
  A. They are malignant neoplasms of the lymphoid tissues.
  B. ALL is the most common malignant disease of childhood.
  C. AML is the most common malignancy in adulthood.
  D. CLL almost always presents with weight loss.

18.11 Which of the following is predominantly a disease of the lymph nodes with the Reed-Sternberg cell and the Pel-Ebstein fever as part of the disease features?
  A. Non-Hodgkin's lymphoma
  B. Hodgkin's disease
  C. CML
  D. Multiple myeloma

18.12 In the case of pancytopenia, which test(s) is essential?
  A. Bone marrow aspirate and biopsy
  B. Peripheral blood smear
  C. Hemoglobin electrophoresis
  D. Immunofixation

18.13 Of the following statements, which is true regarding the basic principles of cancer chemotherapy?
A. The main goal is to induce remission.
B. Chemotherapy is found to be useful in all types of cancer.
C. Large tumors are more sensitive to chemotherapy than small ones.
D. Actively dividing cells are the most sensitive to chemotherapy.

18.14 Which of the following is true regarding the TNM staging system?
A. T stands for the location of the primary tumor.
B. N stands for the presence or absence and extent of regional lymph node metastasis.
C. M stands for the mode of treatment needed.
D. In simultaneous bilateral cancers of paired organs, the highest classification is used.

18.15 Regarding white blood cell counts, a shift to the left refers to
A. White cells congregated on the left side of the slide
B. An increase in the number of early segmented and band neutrophils
C. An increase in basophil count
D. An increase in eosinophil count

18.16 The disorder described as a paradoxic condition in which clotting and hemorrhage occur simultaneously within the vascular system is called
A. Idiopathic thrombocytopenic purpura
B. Von Willebrand disease
C. Polycythemia rubra vera
D. Disseminated intravascular coagulation

18.17 Classic hemophilia, or von Willebrand disease, is a deficiency of
A. Factor VIII
B. Factor IX
C. Factor XII
D. Factor XIII

18.18 Which of the following clotting factors is vitamin K dependent?
  A. Factor III
  B. Factor VI
  C. Factor X
  D. Factor XI

18.19 In sudden massive blood loss, the initial MCV finding would be
  A. >100 fL
  B. 80 to 100 fL
  C. <80 fL
  D. None of the above

18.20 The most abundant protein in the plasma is
  A. Albumin
  B. Globulin
  C. Fibrinogen
  D. Glucose

18.21 Which of the following is **TRUE** regarding the breast?
  A. Scaling around the nipple is a common finding best treated with a steroid cream.
  B. Infections of the breast are common in nonlactating women.
  C. Enlargement of one breast without a distinct mass is not of concern.
  D. Inflammatory breast cancer carries a poor prognosis.

18.22 Breast cancer in the male
  A. With positive lymph nodes, has the same prognostic importance as in females
  B. Should be treated more aggressively than in the female
  C. Accounts for approximately 10% of all breast cancers
  D. Is usually caused by vasectomy

18.23 A unilateral soft and well-defined mass is discovered in the breast of a premenopausal woman. She describes the mass as painful. Which of the following is the best course of action?
  A. Provide immediate surgical referral for a biopsy
  B. Have the patient return in 3 mo for reevaluation
  C. Do an in-office fine-needle aspiration
  D. Refer the patient for a mammogram as soon as possible

18.24 A 64-year-old postmenopausal monogamous woman presents with vaginal bleeding. She is not on hormone replacement therapy. Which of the following is indicated?
  A. Endometrial biopsy
  B. Pelvic ultrasound
  C. Cervical cone biopsy
  D. Abdominal CT

18.25 According to 1997 American Cancer Society estimates, the number one cause of cancer deaths in females is
  A. Lung cancer
  B. Breast cancer
  C. Colon cancer
  D. Pancreatic cancer

18.26 Which of the following is used to help monitor the recurrence of ovarian cancer?
  A. Calcium levels
  B. HCG levels
  C. Pap smears
  D. CA-125 levels

18.27 Testicular cancer commonly
  A. Is associated with cryptorchidism
  B. Occurs after the age of 35
  C. Presents with inguinal lymphadenopathy
  D. Presents in African Americans

18.28 Which of the following is **TRUE** concerning laryngeal cancer?
  A. It is more common in females
  B. It usually presents with hoarseness and cough.

C. The risk is increased by a diet high in riboflavin and iodine.
D. It is most often caused by adenocarcinoma.

18.29 Which of the following cancers has recently started to decline in the U.S.?
A. Breast cancer
B. Prostate cancer
C. Lung cancer
D. Colorectal cancer

18.30 Which of the following may be a presenting complaint in a patient with lung cancer?
A. Headaches
B. Seizures
C. Hemoptysis
D. Any of the above

18.31 If after the history and physical you suspect your patient has lung cancer, what step in the diagnostic workup should you perform next?
A. CA-125
B. Bone scan
C. CT of the chest
D. Chest x-ray

18.32 Which of the following is considered a risk factor for the development of colon cancer?
A. History of lung cancer
B. History of bladder cancer
C. Gardner syndrome
D. Low-fiber diet

18.33 Colon cancer most commonly metastasizes to the
A. Liver
B. Brain
C. Bone
D. Lung

18.34 The presence of the Reed-Sternberg cell is required for the diagnosis of
  A. Non-Hodgkin's lymphoma
  B. Hodgkin's disease
  C. Chronic lymphocytic leukemia
  D. Acute lymphocytic leukemia

18.35 The most common cutaneous malignancy is
  A. Basal cell carcinoma
  B. Squamous cell carcinoma
  C. Malignant melanoma
  D. Clear cell sarcoma

18.36 The most common sites of tumors in the oral cavity are the
  A. Soft palate and tongue
  B. Soft palate and buccal mucosa
  C. Floor of the mouth and soft palate
  D. Floor of the mouth and tongue

18.37 If malignant melanoma occurs in an African American patient, it is most likely to affect the
  A. Arms
  B. Lips
  C. Nails
  D. Scalp

18.38 The most common complaint in patients with metastatic prostate cancer is
  A. Urinary frequency
  B. Urinary urgency
  C. Bone pain
  D. Anorexia

18.39 The most appropriate initial method of detecting prostate cancer is
  A. Transurethral biopsy
  B. Digital rectal exam and PSA
  C. Transrectal ultrasound and PSA
  D. Pelvic CT

18.40 Which two factors are considered synergistic in the development of head and neck cancers?
A. Tobacco and riboflavin
B. Nicotine and menthol
C. Tobacco and peppermint
D. Alcohol and tobacco

18.41 Staging of malignant melanoma is based on
A. Color
B. Thickness
C. Location
D. Surface area

18.42 Multiple myeloma
A. Is the most common primary neoplasm of bone
B. Occurs most often in the second and third decades of life
C. Most often presents as weight loss
D. Is characterized by clinical signs including hypocalcemia and anemia

18.43 The most appropriate way to biopsy a suspected malignant melanoma is
A. Shave biopsy
B. Electrodesiccation
C. Curettage
D. Excisional biopsy

18.44 Which of the following is true concerning bladder cancer?
A. The classic symptom is gross painless hematuria.
B. It occurs more often in females.
C. It is caused by multiple urinary tract infections.
D. It usually occurs in the fourth and fifth decades of life.

18.45 Which of the following is the classic diagnostic triad for pancreatic cancer?
A. Weight loss, jaundice, abdominal pain
B. Abdominal pain, diabetes, jaundice
C. Migrating thrombophlebitis, weight loss, abdominal pain
D. Diabetes, jaundice, weight loss
E. Depression, diabetes, abdominal pain

18.46 Which of the following is **TRUE** regarding thyroid cancer?
A. It is highly malignant with a very poor survival rate.
B. It is most commonly adenocarcinoma.
C. It may present as hoarseness.
D. It is more common in men.

18.47 Which of the following is **TRUE** concerning gastric carcinoma?
A. The incidence is higher in the U.S. than in Japan.
B. Infection with *Helicobacter pylori* is a risk factor.
C. It usually presents with a sudden onset of severe abdominal pain radiating to the back.
D. The primary treatment modality is chemotherapy.

18.48 A 56-year-old farm worker presents with a nonhealing ulceration on his lower lip. Which of the following is the most likely diagnosis?
A. Squamous cell carcinoma
B. Basal cell carcinoma
C. Melanoma
D. Human papillomavirus

18.49 Which of the following is **TRUE** concerning primary brain tumors?
A. They typically metastasize to lung and bone.
B. They are most often caused by ionizing radiation.
C. They often present with weight loss.
D. MRI with contrast is the most valuable diagnostic test.

18.50 Which of the following is considered a risk factor for the development of cervical cancer?
A. Infection with herpes simplex virus type I
B. Infection with human papillomavirus type 16
C. High socioeconomic status
D. Nulliparity

Hematology and Oncology

Answers and Discussion

18.1 (A) Fatigue would be expected, even though it may be very subtle. Other symptoms may occur depending on the specific reason for the anemia. (*1, pp 204–205*)

18.2 (A) NSAID use may cause gastrointestinal bleeding resulting in iron-deficiency anemia especially in the elderly. Koilonychia or spooning of the nails is seen in severe anemia. Anemia is characterized by a low MCV, microcytosis, and hypochromia. (*1, p 210*)

18.3 (D) The reticulocyte count is the initial test performed (simultaneously with the microscopic exam of a peripheral blood smear) to determine the status of erythropoiesis. (*1, p 206*)

18.4 (B) The serum vitamin B_{12} level should be checked in such a patient. (*1, p 212*)

18.5 (C) Pernicious anemia is most likely. Sickle cell anemia and thalassemia major anemias cause a reduction of life span. Iron deficiency would not cause macrocytosis. (*1, p 212*)

18.6 (B) The diagnosis is likely if irreversibly sickled RBCs are present. (*1, p 209*)

18.7 (A) Patients with sickle cell trait usually report no symptoms other than painless hematuria. (*1, p 209*)

18.8 (A) The basic defect of the thalassemia genes is decreased production of a specific globin chain. (*1, pp 206–207*)

18.9 (D) The Philadelphia chromosome represents a translocation between chromosomes 9 and 22 and is a classic feature of chronic myelocytic leukemia (CML). (*2, p 490*)

18.10 (B) Leukemias are malignant neoplasms of the hematopoietic tissues. Acute lymphoblastic leukemia (ALL) is the most common acute leukemia of childhood. (*3, pp 318–337*)

18.11 (B) Hodgkin's disease has various presentations including the Pel-Ebstein fever. Identification of the Reed-Sternberg cell is diagnostic. (*2, p 533*)

18.12 (A) In all unexplained pancytopenias, bone marrow aspiration and biopsy are mandatory. (*2, p 511*)

18.13 (D) The main goal of chemotherapy is to destroy malignant cells without harming normal cells. The most actively dividing cells are most affected. Smaller tumors grow more rapidly than larger ones, and are thus more susceptible to chemotherapy. (*3, p 355*)

18.14 (B) T is the extent of the primary tumor, while M is the presence or absence of distant metastases. In cases involving paired organs, each should be staged separately. (*2, pp 67–68*)

18.15 (B) A shift to the left refers to an increase in the number of immature neutrophils. (*1, p 59*)

18.16 (D) Disseminated intravascular coagulation is a coagulopathy acquired from a variety of causes including infections, cancer, trauma, shock, liver disease, pregnancy, and others. (*5, pp 978–979*)

18.17 (A) In most cases of classic hemophilia (or hemophilia A), factor VIII is quantitatively reduced. (*4, p 93*)

18.18 (C) Factors II, VII, IX, and X require vitamin K for synthesis. (*6, p 367*)

18.19 (B) The initial or early finding in sudden massive blood loss is a normal MCV (80 to 100 fL) or normocytic anemia. (*6, p 376*)

18.20 (A) Albumin is the most abundant protein. Glucose is a carbohydrate. (*6, p 358*)

18.21 (D) Paget's disease, a neoplastic process around the nipple, may look innocent. Breast enlargement even without a mass should be evaluated. Infections of the breast are rare in nonlactating women. (*2, p 203*)

18.22 (A) The natural history and treatment of cancer of the male breast are nearly identical to those in the female. The incidence of this cancer is only 1% of breast cancers. (*2, p 217*)

18.23 (C) Fine-needle aspiration is the best course of action as the lesion is most likely cystic. Withdrawn fluid should be sent for cytology, but this course of action may also be curative. (*7, p 498*)

18.24 (A) Any postmenopausal patient not on hormone replacement therapy who presents with vaginal bleeding should have an endometrial biopsy to rule out cancer. (*3, pp 234–235*)

18.25 (A) Lung cancer has surpassed breast cancer in death rates even though breast cancer still occurs more often. This is presumably due to increased smoking rates in females. (*3, p 10*)

18.26 (D) CA-125 is useful for monitoring the recurrence of and not for screening of ovarian cancer. (*3, pp 243–244*)

18.27 (A) Testicular cancer is most common in whites between the ages of 25 and 35, and in those with a family history of testicular cancer. Cryptorchidism is the best-documented risk factor for testicular cancer. (*3, pp 176–177*)

18.28 (B) Laryngeal cancer is more common in men. It is most often of the squamous cell type. Diets rich in nitrosamines and deficient in vitamin C increase the risk of laryngeal cancer. (*3, p 443*)

18.29 (D) The lung cancer rate is increasing dramatically, presumably because of the increase in the number of female smokers and the latency period. Prostate and breast cancer rates are still rising, presumably because of better diagnostics. Colorectal cancer is decreasing in the U.S. (*3, pp 15–18*)

18.30 (D) Many presentations are possible, depending on the location of the primary tumor and the site(s) of metastasis. (*3, pp 61–63*)

18.31 (D) Chest x-ray is the most appropriate next step. (*3, pp 70–71*)

18.32 (E) Gardner syndrome, a familial polyposis syndrome, is a risk factor. A low- or high-fiber diet has not correlated well with risk. (*3, pp 143–145*)

18.33 (A) Colorectal cancer is spread by contiguous invasion or via lymphatic channels to the liver. (*3, p 150*)

18.34 (B) The giant cell known as the R-S cell is required for the diagnosis of Hodgkin's disease. (*2, p 451*)

18.35 (A) Basal cell carcinoma is the most common cutaneous malignancy. UVB light is the most implicated causative factor. (*2, p 330*)

18.36 (D) The floor of the mouth and the tongue are the most common sites of tumors in the oral cavity. Tobacco use is the major risk factor. (*2, p 369*)

18.37 (C) Acral lentiginous melanoma, rarely found in Caucasians, accounts for 35% to 60% of melanomas in dark-skinned persons. Look for lesions on the palms, soles, and nailbeds. (*3, p 287; 2, p 305*)

18.38 (C) Patients with metastases to the bone most commonly complain of bone pain. (*2, p 315*)

18.39 (B) The digital rectal exam (DRE) is the easiest and most cost-effective test for prostate cancer. It should be performed yearly after the age of 40. The posterior surfaces of the lateral lobes, where the cancer begins most often, are easily palpated. DRE combined with PSA is optimal. Abnormalities of either require further evaluation. (*3, p 160*)

18.40 (D) Tobacco use and alcohol abuse constitute a combination that promotes the development of malignant growths. (*2, p 358*)

18.41 (B) Staging of malignant melanoma is based on microscopic assessment of thickness. (*2, pp 305–306*)

18.42 (A) Multiple myeloma occurs most often in men in the sixth and seventh decades of life. The usual presenting symptom is bone pain. Clinically, the disease presents with anemia, hypercalcemia, renal insufficiency, and recurrent infections. (*3, pp 264–265*)

18.43 (D) Full-thickness excisional biopsy with extended margins is most appropriate for suspected malignant melanoma. The full thickness is necessary to determine both stage and prognosis. (*3, p 288*)

18.44 (A) Bladder cancer occurs more often in men ages 60 to 70. The cause is unknown, but cigarette smoking and chemical exposure are suspected, in addition to genetic mechanisms. (*3, pp 168–169*)

18.45 (A) Abdominal pain, jaundice, and weight loss constitute the classic triad for pancreatic cancer. Other symptoms may include migrating thrombophlebitis and depression. Diabetes may occur months before the diagnosis. (*3, pp 114–115*)

18.46 (C) Thyroid cancer may present with hoarseness if the tumor is pressing on the recurrent laryngeal nerve. This cancer has a high survival rate if caught early. It is usually of the papillary or mixed papillary-follicular type. (*3, pp 98–100*)

18.47 (B)   Infection with *H. pylori* is considered a risk factor for gastric cancer. The incidence of gastric cancer is much higher in Japan than in the U.S. The symptoms are usually vague and include abdominal pain and bloating. The primary treatment modality is surgery. (*3, pp 133–135*)

18.48 (B)   Squamous cell carcinoma is the most likely diagnosis. Exposure to the sun is a major risk factor, and farm workers are at very high risk for this type of cancer. (*3, p 48*)

18.49 (D)   MRI with contrast is the best modality to determine the presence of a tumor in the brain. (*3, p 30*)

18.50 (B)   HPV type 16 is considered a high risk, along with many other risk factors. (*3, p 187*)

References

1. Astuto A, Chou PP, Otero D, et al: Gynecology. In: Rucker LM (ed): *Essentials of Adult Ambulatory Care,* Baltimore, Williams & Wilkins, 1997.

2. Murphy GP, Lawrence W Jr, Lenhard RE Jr (eds): *American Cancer Society Textbook of Clinical Oncology,* 2/e, American Cancer Society, 1995.

3. Boyer KL, Kantarjian H: Acute and chronic leukemias—A concise review. In: Boyer KL, Ford MB, Judkins AF, et al (eds): *Primary Care Oncology,* Philadelphia, Saunders, 1999.

4. Ravel R: *Clinical Laboratory Medicine,* 6/e, St. Louis, Mosby, 1995.

5. Eberst ME: Acquired bleeding disorders. In: Tintinalli JE, Kelen GD, Stapczynski (eds): *Emergency Medicine: A Comprehensive Study Guide,* 4/e, New York, McGraw-Hill, 2000.

6. Pagana KD, Pagana TJ: *Mosby's Manual of Diagnostic and Laboratory Tests,* St. Louis, Mosby, 1998.

7. Sloane PD, et al (eds): *Essentials of Family Medicine,* Baltimore, Williams & Wilkins, 1998.

19

Substance Abuse and Psychopharmacology

Jeff Baker, PhD

DIRECTIONS (Questions 19.1–19.32): Each of the numbered items or incomplete statements in this chapter is followed by answers or completions of the statement. Select the **one** lettered answer or completion that is **best** in each case.

19.1 According to the DSM-IV, which is **NOT** a criterion for substance dependence?

A. There is evidence of familial patterns of substance abuse or dependence (especially by parents or full siblings).

B. Important social, occupational, or recreational activities are given up or reduced because of substance abuse.

C. There is a persistent desire or unsuccessful efforts to cut down or to control the use of the substance.

D. Tolerance has developed, as defined by a need for markedly increased amounts of the substance to achieve intoxication or the desired effect.

19.2 Which of the following has the lowest abuse potential?

A. Barbiturates

B. Opium

C. Cocaine

D. Buspirone
E. Amphetamines

19.3 Which of the following is **NOT** a psychiatric syndrome of AIDS?
A. Dementia
B. Anxiety disorders
C. Depressive disorders
D. Financial stress

19.4 Which is not a DSM-IV diagnostic criterion for Intermittent Explosive Disorder?
A. Recurrent failure to resist impulses to steal objects
B. Several discrete episodes of failure to resist aggressive impulses that result in serious assaultive acts or destruction of property
C. Degree of aggressiveness expressed during episodes that is grossly out of proportion to any precipitating psychosocial stressors
D. Aggressive episodes not better accounted for by an antisocial personality disorder
E. Aggressive episodes not better accounted for by a borderline personality disorder

19.5 All of the following are diagnostic criteria for cocaine intoxication **EXCEPT**
A. Recent use of cocaine
B. Clinically significant maladaptive behavioral or psychological changes that develop during or shortly after the use of cocaine
C. History of use and abuse of cocaine by family and friends
D. Elevated or lowered blood pressure
E. Muscular weakness, respiratory depression, chest pain, or cardiac arrhythmias

19.6 Which of the following causes of decreased libido need **NOT** be investigated at the initial visit?
A. Medication and/or substance use
B. Posttraumatic stress disorder
C. Presence of a chronic medical condition
D. Unresolved issues of love in childhood
E. Learned sexual information and behaviors

19.7 All of the following are conditions that may reduce patient adherence to treatment with psychotropic agents **EXCEPT**
   A. Complex therapeutic regimen
   B. Minimal adverse drug reactions
   C. Slow onset of beneficial effects
   D. Financial hardships and/or conflicting obligations of time or money
   E. Involvement of multiple clinicians

19.8 Psychotropic—particularly serotonergic—agents may be associated with impairment of
   A. Libido
   B. Ejaculation
   C. Erection
   D. Female orgasm
   E. All of the above

19.9 Buspirone (BuSpar), the first clinically available azaspirone in the United States, is approved for the treatment of
   A. Anxiety disorders
   B. Eating disorders
   C. Sexual disorders
   D. Depressive disorders

19.10 All the following disorders are currently being treated with selective serotonin reuptake inhibitors (SSRIs) **EXCEPT**
   A. Depression
   B. Eating disorders
   C. Panic disorder
   D. Sexual desire disorders
   E. Obsessive-compulsive disorders

19.11 For depression, the initial dose of fluoxetine (Prozac) is usually 20 mg PO qd, usually given in the morning because insomnia is a potential adverse drug reaction. The maximum daily dosage recommended by the manufacturer is 80 mg because higher doses may result in
   A. Intense anxiety
   B. Seizures
   C. Heart failure

D. Addiction problems
E. Euphoria

19.12 Neuroleptic-induced parkinsonism is characterized principally by
A. Stuttering, heart palpitations, and anxiety
B. Resting tremor, rigidity, and bradykinesia
C. Momentary resting followed by the softening of muscles until anxious
D. Spontaneous speech characterized by thickening of the tongue
E. All of the above

19.13 All the following are special factors to consider when prescribing venlafaxine (Effexor) **EXCEPT**
A. Absence of side effects
B. Energizing effect
C. Rapid onset
D. Effectiveness for depression

19.14 All of the following are considerations when prescribing nefazodone (Serzone) **EXCEPT**
A. Expense
B. Excellent tolerability
C. Ease of overdose
D. Necessity for titration

19.15 All of the following are special factors in prescribing Remeron **EXCEPT**
A. Use for chronic pain
B. Use as an anxiolytic, anti-panic drug
C. Lack of weight gain
D. Limited sexual dysfunction

19.16 All of the following are antiabuse medications **EXCEPT**
A. Antabuse
B. Methadone
C. ReVia
D. Opium

19.17 Which is **NOT** a DSM-IV criterion for pedophilia?
A. It lasts for at least 6 mo.
B. It involves recurrent, intense sexual fantasies, sexual urges, or behaviors involving sexual activity with a prepubescent child or children.
C. The fantasies and sexual urges are well controlled with alcohol use.
D. The fantasies and sexual urges cause considerable distress or impairment in social, occupational, or other important areas of functioning.
E. The person (perpetrator) is at least 16 years old, and at least 5 years older than the child or children.

19.18 All of the following are myths regarding alcoholism treatment **EXCEPT**
A. Nothing works.
B. There is one particular approach that is superior to all others.
C. Eclecticism is the only approach proven effective.
D. All treatment approaches work about equally well.
E. Trial and error reigns in alcoholism treatment programs.

19.19 Which of the following is **NOT** a model of alcoholism treatment?
A. Temperance
B. American disease
C. Educational
D. Shock treatment
E. Social learning

19.20 All the following statements are true of alcoholism treatment and of reduction in drinking behaviors **EXCEPT**
A. Deemphasis on labels and acceptance of the alcoholism label is seen as unnecessary for change to occur.
B. The problem drinker must be enabled by helping him or her to identify excuses for his or her drinking behaviors.
C. Emphasis must be placed on personal choice regarding future use of alcohol and other drugs.
D. The health care practitioner conducts an objective evaluation, but focuses on eliciting the client's own concerns.
E. Resistance by the problem drinker is met with reflection.

19.21 Chronic alcohol abuse takes its toll on the body's organ systems. The following are all **TRUE** statements **EXCEPT**

A. Comprehensive intake and follow-up evaluation includes assessment of the patient's physical health.

B. It is quite possible for a person to be drinking in a manner that damages the body without showing major life problems or dependence symptoms.

C. Individuals with diagnosable alcohol abuse or dependence never show concomitant problems as well.

D. A serum chemistry panel can be obtained from a small blood sample, and may reflect alcohol-related abnormalities.

E. Liver enzymes such as serum glutamic-oxaloacetic transaminase (SGOT) and gamma glutamyl transpeptidase (GGT) should be included in a serum chemistry panel.

19.22 All the following are important concepts in the self-control training model of alcohol abuse treatment **EXCEPT**

A. Setting limits on how many drinks one will have and moving from stronger to weaker drinks

B. Refusing drinks when one is offered additional drinks

C. Setting up a reward system for success

D. Spending more time alone and avoiding even important support systems

E. Identifying patterns in one's drinking behaviors

19.23 The following are all part of the Twelve Steps of Alcoholics Anonymous **EXCEPT**

A. We admitted we were powerless over alcohol—that our lives had become unmanageable.

B. Came to believe that a Power greater than ourselves could restore us to sanity.

C. Money and power is our best solution to refocus our thoughts and energy.

D. Made a searching and fearless moral inventory of ourselves.

E. Made a list of all persons we had harmed, and became willing to make amends to them all.

19.24 The following are all substances that have been abused
EXCEPT
  A. Nitrous oxide
  B. Nitrite inhalants
  C. Anabolic steroids
  D. Catnip
  E. Beetle juice

19.25 Carbamazepine (Tegretol) is an iminodibenzyl drug that is
structurally similar to imipramine (Tofranil) and is approved
for use in the United States to treat
  A. Temporal lobe epilepsy
  B. General epilepsy
  C. Trigeminal neuralgia
  D. All of the above
  E. A and B only

19.26 The manufacturer recall of flenfluramine (Pondimin) and
desfenfluramine (Redux) in September 1997 occurred be-
cause
  A. Companies were concerned about the legal and ethical
     consequences of continuing to market the drugs.
  B. The drugs were associated with serious heart and lung
     problems.
  C. Consumers were no longer interested in these medica-
     tions.
  D. The drug companies were no longer able to make money
     on these drugs.
  E. All of the above

19.27 Hypericum, which is currently undergoing clinical research
trials for effectiveness in comparison to imipramine, is the
principal component of
  A. St. John's wort
  B. Ginkgo biloba
  C. Saw palmetto
  D. Damania
  E. Ginseng

19.28 Which of the following is the most commonly used short-term and prophylactic treatment for Bipolar I Disorder?
A. Lithium
B. Haloperidol
C. Barbiturates
D. Amphetamines
E. Clonidine

19.29 Methadone is used in psychiatry primarily for
A. Hyperactivity
B. Anxiety disorders
C. Detoxification
D. Sexual aversion disorders

19.30 Which of the following would **NOT** be prescribed as an antipsychotic if extrapyramidal side effects were a concern?
A. Haloperidol (Haldol)
B. Clozapine (Clozaril)
C. Risperidone (Risperidol)
D. Sertindole

19.31 All of the following are complications of MAO inhibitors **EXCEPT**
A. Orthostatic hypotension
B. Weight gain
C. Hypersexuality
D. Insomnia

19.32 All of the following are considered true regarding electro-convulsive therapy (ECT) **EXCEPT**
A. It is one of the most effective and least understood treatments in psychiatry.
B. It is considered safe and effective for treatment of patients with depressive disorders.
C. It is underused because of widespread misinformation and inflammatory information in the media.
D. It has never been shown to be a safe and effective therapy.
E. It may relieve severe depression within 1 wk, but the full benefit requires several treatments over a few weeks.

Substance Abuse and Psychopharmacology

Answers and Discussion

19.1 (B)ᴬ   Although it may be common to find that family members have also abused substances, it is not a criterion of the DSM-IV. (*1, p 377*)

anti-anxiety

19.2 (D)   Buspirone is one of the more effective medications to give to individuals who have a history of substance abuse, as it has a low addictive potential. (*1, pp 1004–1005*)

19.3 (E)   Although financial stress is many times an outcome in individuals with AIDS, it is not a psychiatric syndrome that accompanies AIDS. (*1, pp 367–369*)

19.4 (A)   Stealing is not part of the diagnostic criteria for Intermittent Explosive Disorder. (*1, pp 761–763*)

19.5 (C)   It is not unfamiliar for friends and family members to also be users of cocaine, but it is not one of the diagnostic criteria for cocaine intoxication. (*1, p 423*)

19.6 (D)   Unresolved issues of love in childhood may have something to do with hyposexual functioning, but are not a criterion that should be fully investigated until the other factors are ruled out, especially in the initial exam. (*1*, *pp 684–685*)

19.7 (B) A lack of side effects would be one of the best motivators for adherence to a medication. Many individuals discontinue psychopharmacology due to unwanted side effects. (*1*, *p 956*)

19.8 (E) All of the side effects mentioned are common with serotonergic drug interventions. (*1*, *p 1072*)

19.9 (A) BuSpar and other hypnotics have practically eliminated the use of barbiturates for the treatment of anxiety. BuSpar has a lower abuse potential, higher therapeutic index, and lack of hepatic enzyme induction. (*1*, *pp 1004–1006*)

19.10 (D) Sexual desire is usually inhibited by the SSRIs. (*1*, *pp 684–685*)

19.11 (B) The highest recommended dose of fluoxetine (Prozac) is 80 mg. At higher levels individuals can experience seizures. (*1*, *pp 1087–1088*)

19.12 (B) Neuroleptic-induced parkinsonism is characterized principally by the triad of resting tremor, rigidity, and bradykinesia (referred to in the DSM-IV as akinesia). The typical parkinsonian tremor oscillates at a steady rate of 3 to 6 cycles per second, and it may be suppressed by intended movement. Rigidity is a disorder of muscle tone—that is, the degree of underlying tension involuntarily present in the muscles. (*1*, *pp 957–958*)

19.13 (A) Effexor has a high frequency of side effects and must be carefully monitored by the health care practitioner. (*1*, *pp 1081–1083*)

19.14 (C) Serzone is one of the safer medications regarding overdose. (*1*, *pp 1067–1069*)

19.15 (C) Weight gain is one of the unfortunate side effects of Remeron. (*1*, *pp 1057–1059*)

19.16 (D) Opium has a high addiction probability and would not be a good medication to give someone with risks for addictive factors. (*1, p 439*)

19.17 (C) Many times alcohol appears to be part of child sexual abuse, as it may lower inhibitions and reduce social control of potential perpetrators. (*1, pp 397–399*)

19.18 (E) Trial and error reigns as the only truth among these myths. There is no particular treatment that works better than others, yet some treatment programs are more effective than others in certain cases. (*2, p 109*)

19.19 (D) All of the models listed are treatment programs for alcoholism except the shock treatment model. It has been suggested but never put forth as a formidable model for treatment and would never be approved by an institutional review board in the ethical treatment of human subjects. (*2, pp 128–138*)

19.20 (B) Enabling the problem drinker to find additional excuses would not be an effective way of getting the individual to examine the real issues and consequences in problem drinking. Resistance is better met with simple reflection of what the problem drinker is stating and then disputing the irrational beliefs behind those behaviors. (*2, p 75*)

19.21 (C) Individuals frequently show concomitant problems when alcoholism is suspected. These might include other impulsive behaviors or psychosocial concerns such as strained interpersonal relationships, financial stressors, poor work history, and absenteeism. (*2, p 183*)

19.22 (D) Spending time alone is not a very wise strategy for an individual seeking to control his or her drinking. It is important to spend time with positive support systems. Avoiding drinking buddies might assist in the self-control training program. (*2, p 110*)

19.23 (C) Money and power are many times highly correlated with drinking problems. Sometimes the pursuit of both of these goals leads people to drink, and sometimes the lack of those resources leads people to use alcohol to soothe themselves. (*2, p 3*)

19.24 (E) *Beetlejuice* was a popular movie, and there is no indication it is a substance that has been abused. All of the other materials have been used in substance abuse. (*1, p 389*)

19.25 (D) Tegretol has been approved to treat temporal lobe epilepsy, general epilepsy, and trigeminal neuralgia. (*1, pp 1008–1014*)

19.26 (B) Studies indicated that Pondimin and Redux had possible serious side effects related to severe heart and lung problems. (*1, pp 1042–1044*)

19.27 (A) Hypericum is a principal component of St. John's wort and is currently being studied for its role in treating depression. (*1, p 1126*)

19.28 (A) Lithium is the most commonly used treatment for bipolar disorders. (*1, pp 1046–1055*)

19.29 (C) Methadone is used commonly in the detoxification of substance abuse, primarily heroin abuse. It is currently also being used in the treatment of chronic pain. (*1, pp 1055–1057*)

19.30 (A) Haldol has the most extrapyramidal effects of all of the drugs listed. (*1, p 1029*)

19.31 (C) Hypersexuality is not a side effect of MAO inhibitors. Typically, the concern is hyposexuality. (*1, pp 1059–1064*)

19.32 (D) ECT has been shown to be a safe and effective treatment for depression. (*1, pp 1115–1122*)

References

1. Kaplan HI, Sadock BJ: *Synopsis of Psychiatry: Behavioral Sciences/Clinical Psychiatry,* 8/e, Baltimore, Williams & Wilkins, 1998.

2. Hester RK, Miller WR (eds): *Handbook of Alcoholism: Treatment Approaches: Effective Alternatives,* 2/e, New York, Pergamon, 1989.

20

Emergency Medicine

Frances Coulson, MS, PA-C

DIRECTIONS (Questions 20.1–20.80): Each of the numbered items or incomplete statements in this chapter is followed by answers or completions of the statement. Select the **one** lettered answer or completion that is **best** in each case.

20.1 The most common symptoms of spontaneous pneumothorax are
   A. Chest pain and dyspnea
   B. Anterior chest pain and hemoptysis
   C. Cough and dyspnea
   D. Wheezing and hemoptysis

20.2 Which of the following would be found in a case of tension pneumothorax?
   A. Hypertension and flattened neck veins
   B. Hyperresonance on the side opposite the pneumothorax
   C. Deviation of the trachea toward the side of the pneumothorax
   D. Cyanosis and severe dyspnea

20.3 The appropriate first-line care for a patient with a tension pneumothorax is
  A. A confirmatory CXR to determine the correct diagnosis prior to intervening
  B. Immediate endotracheal intubation to provide an adequate airway
  C. An emergency thoracotomy for decompression
  D. Positive-pressure ventilation with a demand valve

20.4 On physical exam, a patient experiencing an asthmatic attack may exhibit which of the following?
  A. Lung fields dull to percussion
  B. Prolonged inspiratory phase
  C. Hemoptysis
  D. Expiratory wheezes

20.5 Which of the following may be a cause of wheezing in the adult patient?
  A. CHF
  B. Bronchogenic carcinoma
  C. Vocal cord dysfunction
  D. All of the above

20.6 A 52-year-old patient presents with acute, steady, severe retrosternal chest pain that radiates to the back. The pain worsens with chest motion. On exam, a pericardial friction rub is auscultated. This presentation is most consistent with
  A. AMI
  B. Esophageal colic
  C. Pneumonia
  D. Pericarditis

20.7 A 25-year-old, 32-wk-pregnant woman presents with right upper quadrant (RUQ) pain, nausea, and vomiting. Which of the following is the most likely diagnosis?
  A. Hyperemesis gravidarum
  B. Appendicitis
  C. Colitis
  D. Pulmonary embolism

20.8 A 78-year-old nursing home patient presents with feculent vomiting and abdominal bloating. Which of the following is most likely?
A. Mesenteric ischemia
B. Diverticulitis
C. Bowel obstruction
D. Cholecystitis

20.9 The finding considered diagnostic of intestinal obstruction on x-ray is
A. Free air under the diaphragm
B. Air-fluid levels
C. Gas pattern throughout the large intestine
D. Fat pad sign

20.10 Four adults go on a retreat in the mountains of Colorado. After flying by private plane, they reach Pike's Peak (approximately 14,000 ft). After having a few drinks, they turn in for the night. Upon awakening, one individual complains of HA, N/V, SOB, and weakness. The others note his facial swelling and general irritability. Which of the following is the most appropriate treatment?
A. Lorazepam 2 mg PO
B. Increased intake of fluids
C. Descent and oxygen
D. Furosemide 40 mg IV

20.11 Which of the following would **NOT** be expected in decompression sickness?
A. Hematemesis
B. Rash
C. Subcutaneous emphysema
D. Leg paresthesias

20.12 A 35-year-old man arrives in the ED complaining of severe knee and shoulder pain and bilateral lower extremity paresthesias. You learn that earlier in the day he was in Cancun, where he jogged 5 mi, then went scuba diving and spearfished for the entire afternoon in 80 ft of water. He then caught an airplane back to the States in the evening. When asked about whether he followed the dive table, he acts confused about the question. What treatment is appropriate?
A. Joint aspiration for nitrogen crystals
B. Air transport to the nearest level I trauma center
C. IV D5W and furosemide 40 mg IV
D. High-flow oxygen and recompression

20.13 For a patient in cardiopulmonary arrest presenting with ventricular tachycardia, what is the most definitive treatment according to ACLS guidelines?
A. CPR
B. 100% oxygen
C. Defibrillation
D. Synchronized cardioversion
E. Epinephrine

20.14 Which of the following can be a cause of pulseless electrical activity?
A. Hypervolemia
B. Cardiac tamponade
C. Simple pneumothorax
D. Pulmonary edema

20.15 In a patient presenting with chest pain, diaphoresis, decreased level of consciousness, and ventricular tachycardia, which of the following is the most appropriate treatment?
A. Verapamil 2.5 mg IV
B. Lidocaine 1 mg/kg IV
C. Adenosine 6 mg rapid IVP
D. Synchronized cardioversion

20.16 Your patient is a 22-year-old man who has overdosed on amitriptyline. He most likely will present with

    A. Dysrhythmias
    B. Vomiting
    C. Renal failure
    D. Liver failure

20.17 Four victims were simultaneously struck by lightning; only one is in cardiopulmonary arrest (the others are unconscious but breathing). What should you do first if you are the only rescuer?
    A. Initiate CPR on the patient in arrest.
    B. Give care to the survivors in standing with the traditional triage system.
    C. Find help prior to initiating any care.
    D. Drag all patients to a safe area.

20.18 An adult patient suffers second-degree steam burns to the entire front of his trunk, the anterior surface of his right arm, and his entire right leg. What percentage of the body has been burned?
    A. 40.5%
    B. 45%
    C. 36%
    D. 38%

20.19 Assuming no other injuries are present, which of the following treatments should be considered for the burn patient in question 20.18?
    A. Chilled sheets applied to stop the burn
    B. Tetanus toxoid booster
    C. Full assessment of all burns prior to pain control
    D. Placement of central lines for fluid resuscitation

20.20 Which of the following is **TRUE** concerning electricity?
    A. Alternating current at 60 cycles/s is less dangerous than direct current of the same amperage.
    B. In general, the higher the voltage, the more severe the injury.
    C. Muscles and nerves are more resistant to the flow of electricity than are bone and skin.
    D. Most electrical injuries occur to children under the age of 6 years.

20.21 Alkali burns cause more tissue damage than do acids because alkali produce
A. Coagulation necrosis
B. Liquefaction necrosis
C. Protein denaturation
D. An exothermic reaction

20.22 In almost all chemical burns, whether to skin or eyes, the cornerstone of initial treatment is
A. Careful identification of the offending agent
B. A search for the appropriate neutralizing agent
C. Hydrotherapy
D. Analgesics

20.23 A 72-year-old man presents to the ED complaining of a syncopal episode earlier in the day. Which of the following is the most appropriate test for the initial workup?
A. Sedimentation rate
B. ECG
C. Urine drug test
D. MRI of the head

20.24 Rapid-onset syncope in the elderly patient in a seated or lying position is most likely due to
A. Vasovagal syncope
B. Seizure disorder
C. Hyperventilation
D. Cardiac disease

20.25 A 32-year-old woman has ingested home-canned green beans and is experiencing nausea and vomiting. She also complains of dry mouth and difficulty urinating. You suspect food poisoning. You notice general weakness and ptosis. What is the most likely offending agent?
A. *Clostridium difficile*
B. *Clostridium botulinum*
C. *Clostridium perfringens*
D. *Clostridium jejuni*

20.26 What would you find on chest x-ray of a patient with pneumothorax?

A. Kerley B lines
B. Enlarged mediastinum with a flattened diaphragm
C. Blunting of the costophrenic angles
D. Hyperlucency with lack of lung markings at the periphery

20.27 Which of the following is the appropriate management of a cat bite to the hand?
A. Primary wound closure of all wounds
B. Prophylactic antibiotics
C. Tetanus immune globulin if prophylaxis is older than 3 years
D. Debridement of puncture wounds to enhance primary closure

20.28 A 67-year-old woman presents to the ED with trismus, risus sardonicus, a rigid abdominal wall, and hyperreflexia. Her spouse states she has been complaining of neck and jaw stiffness and back and abdominal pain, and that she sustained a small laceration on her hand about 1 wk earlier. The patient is normally very active and spends much time in her garden. She takes no medications and has not seen a doctor in many years. What is the most likely cause of this patient's symptoms?
A. *C. botulinum*
B. *Clostridium tetani*
C. Subarachnoid hemorrhage
D. Meningitis

20.29 A painter has suffered a high-pressure paint injection injury to his left hand. Which of the following is most appropriate?
A. Flushing the wound with saline and primary closure
B. Secondary closure of the hand and splinting
C. Flushing with carbon tetrachloride, then splinting
D. Referral to a hand surgeon

20.30 Which of the following is the best diagnostic test in a patient with positive Brudzinski and Kernig signs?
A. CT of the head
B. CSF analysis
C. CBC
D. PT and PTT

20.31 It is midsummer in New York. A 67-year-old man is brought unconscious to the ED. His skin is hot and dry. He is disheveled, smells heavily of alcohol, and has blood on his lips. His core temperature is 41°C. Your differential should include
  A. Heat stroke
  B. Alcohol withdrawal
  C. Acute salicylate intoxication
  D. All of the above

20.32 Which technique is considered easiest and most effective in cooling a hyperthermic patient?
  A. Cold peritoneal lavage
  B. Cold gastric lavage
  C. Cold water immersion
  D. Evaporative cooling

20.33 A lawn maintenance supervisor presents to your clinic complaining of an insect bite to his neck, tightness in his throat, and difficulty breathing. You notice stridor and dyspnea. Which is the most appropriate initial treatment?
  A. Identification of the offending agent
  B. Cold packs to the bite site
  C. 0.3 to 0.5 mL of 1:1000 epinephrine SQ
  D. Diphenhydramine (Benadryl) 50 mg PO

20.34 Which of the following is **TRUE** regarding hypothermia?
  A. It most often affects those intoxicated with drugs or alcohol.
  B. Cold water immersion causes slower heat loss than does convection.
  C. Ventricular fibrillation is likely in mild hypothermia.
  D. The diagnosis of hypothermia is obvious.

20.35 Which of the following requires urgent intervention in a patient complaining of low back pain?
  A. Loss of bladder control
  B. Palpable paraspinal muscle spasm

C. Slow onset of nonradiating pain
D. Pain aggravated by bending

20.36 The most appropriate first aid treatment for rattlesnake envenomation is
A. Ice water immersion of the injury site
B. Tourniquet to the affected limb
C. Immobilization of the affected limb
D. Cuts placed through the fang marks and application of suction

20.37 Acute compartment syndrome should be suspected if the patient has
A. Severe pain in the extremity
B. A loose-fitting cast
C. Bounding pulses in the extremity
D. Hyperesthesia in the affected extremity

20.38 A patient with a history of small cell carcinoma of the lung presents with facial swelling and telangiectasias, headache, and bilateral papilledema. You should
A. Perform a lumbar puncture
B. Place the patient in the Trendelenburg position
C. Initiate large-bore IVs of normal saline
D. Administer diuretics and glucocorticoids

20.39 Which of the following would lead to the diagnosis of loxoscelism (sequelae from the bite of a brown recluse spider)?
A. Large hairy brown spider with thick legs brought in with the patient
B. Circumoral paresthesias
C. Seizures immediately following envenomation
D. Initial local pain and erythema followed by central bleb or pustule

20.40 The reactions to a black widow spider bite may include
A. Large area of pain, erythema, and edema
B. Abdominal rigidity
C. Tissue sloughing in the bite area in 48 to 72 h
D. Hypotension

20.41 A patient with acute epistaxis who is seen after the bleeding has stopped
A. Can be released without further evaluation
B. Should have the site of bleeding identified
C. Should have a PT/PTT drawn even with a normal medical history
D. Should have anterior nasal packing applied

20.42 Which of the following must be considered in the evaluation and treatment of near-drowning victims?
A. Hyperglycemia
B. Status post renal failure
C. Metabolic alkalosis
D. Hypothermia

20.43 A normally healthy individual should be considered at risk for hepatotoxicity if he or she has ingested what amount of acetaminophen?
A. 1400 mg/kg
B. 140 mg/kg
C. 40 mg/kg
D. 4 mg/kg

20.44 What is the antidote for acetaminophen overdose?
A. Acetylcholecysteine
B. Acetaminophate
C. Naloxone
D. *N*-acetylcysteine

20.45 Numerous patients from a crowded and smoke-filled bingo hall present with complaints of nausea, dizziness, throbbing headache, and paresthesias. The most likely cause is
A. Heat exhaustion
B. Claustrophobic neurosis
C. Alcohol intoxication
D. Carbon monoxide exposure

20.46 What is the appropriate treatment in the situation in question 20.45?
  A. 100% oxygen
  B. Benzodiazepines
  C. Acetylation
  D. Amyl nitrate

20.47 In the assessment and management of a patient with possible head injury
  A. A high blood alcohol level rules out a brain injury.
  B. Loss of consciousness indicates the need for a head CT.
  C. Hypotension is a sign of severe head injury.
  D. Deterioration is expected and is managed with IV mannitol.

20.48 A permanent tooth that has become avulsed or knocked out should be
  A. Saved so that the ED practitioner knows it is not in the patient's airway
  B. Soaked in salt water for 2 h, then replaced into the socket
  C. Immediately replaced into its socket after a gentle rinse without touching the root surface
  D. Saved for possible replacement by a dentist

20.49 You suspect a patient has a penetrating injury to the eye. You should not perform
  A. Shiotz tonometry exam
  B. Facial radiographs
  C. Slit-lamp exam
  D. Visual acuity exam

20.50 Which test(s) is considered most accurate in the assessment of a patient for possible intra-abdominal injury following blunt trauma?
  A. KUB and physical exam
  B. Diagnostic peritoneal lavage (DPL) and abdominal CT
  C. NG tube contents and flat and upright abdominal films
  D. UA and DPL

20.51 A 55-year-old patient with a history of HTN presents with low back pain radiating to the abdomen and groin. The right femoral pulse is diminished. The most likely diagnosis is
   A. Dissecting abdominal aortic aneurysm
   B. Mesenteric infarction
   C. Cholelithiasis
   D. Nephrolithiasis

20.52 Which of the following is universally present in patients with mesenteric ischemia or infarction?
   A. Abdominal pain
   B. Vomiting
   C. Diarrhea
   D. Hematochezia

20.53 A patient with Marfan syndrome complains of sudden onset of tearing pain in the chest, migrating to the back. On CXR, he has a widened mediastinum. Which of the following is the most likely diagnosis?
   A. Aortic dissection
   B. Myocardial infarction
   C. Pericarditis
   D. Pulmonary embolus

20.54 Which statement about testicular torsion is **TRUE?**
   A. It usually occurs in men over age 40.
   B. It commonly occurs during exertion.
   C. It should be surgically corrected within 48 h.
   D. It occurs as a result of the "bell clapper" deformity.

20.55 Which is the test of choice to determine testicular torsion?
   A. Ultrasonography
   B. Radionuclide scanning
   C. UA
   D. Doppler exam for blood flow

20.56 A victim of a motor vehicle accident (MVA) (small car into a tree) is brought to the ED by private vehicle. Femoral pulses are palpable, but radial pulses are not. What may be assumed from this?

A. An aortic tear is preventing blood flow to the arms.
B. The patient has a systolic blood pressure of at least 70.
C. The patient has no diastolic blood pressure.
D. The patient has a cervical spine injury.

20.57 What would be important to know about the mechanism of injury for the patient in question 20.56?
A. Use of seatbelt
B. Condition of the other passengers
C. Ambient temperature
D. Damage to the patient's vehicle
E. All of the above

20.58 Which of the following is appropriate in the primary survey of a trauma patient?
A. Chest x-ray
B. Splinting of unstable fractures
C. Rectal exam
D. Endotracheal intubation

20.59 What is the definitive treatment for hypovolemia secondary to hemorrhage?
A. Locating the source and stopping the blood loss
B. Infusing large volumes of crystalloids
C. Performing blood transfusions
D. Applying a tourniquet

20.60 In a trauma patient with distended neck veins, which of the following should be considered as the cause?
A. Hypovolemia
B. Cardiac tamponade
C. Head injury
D. Splenic rupture

20.61 In a human bite to the hand, what is the appropriate ED treatment?
A. Thoroughly irrigate and suture the wounds.
B. X-ray, irrigate, and suture the wounds.
C. X-ray and suture the wounds, and use broad-spectrum antibiotics.
D. X-ray and irrigate, use antibiotics, and splint.

20.62 A 23-year-old patient falls onto his knees while playing rugby. He is unable to perform a straight-leg raise. Which of the following is most likely?

A. X-ray will reveal a high-riding patella and surgical consultation is required.

B. X-ray will reveal a torn ACL that requires prompt surgical evaluation.

C. X-ray will reveal a meniscal tear that will heal in 2 to 3 wk.

D. X-ray will reveal a torn lateral collateral ligament requiring immediate surgery.

20.63 A patient presents to the ED with a locked knee. What is the most common cause?

A. Bucket-handle tear of the meniscus

B. ACL rupture

C. Hamstring spasm

D. Dislocated patella

20.64 A victim of an amputation arrives in the ED with the severed part. If you anticipate the possibility of replantation, you should care for the amputated part by

A. Applying antiseptic solution to the wound

B. Using hemostats to stop the bleeding

C. Keeping the wound moist with sterile dressings

D. Packing the severed part in ice water

20.65 A 22-year-old patient presents with acute unilateral soft palate swelling and erythema. On exam, the uvula is pushed to the contralateral side. Which of the following is most likely?

A. Peritonsillar abscess

B. Epiglottitis

C. Mononucleosis

D. Torus palatinus

20.66 During CPR, a patient is intubated and bagged with 100% oxygen. After the patient is moved to the CCU, lung sounds are heard on the right but not the left. What is the most likely problem?

A. Left pneumothorax

B. Tube pushed into the right mainstem bronchus

    C. Right tension pneumothorax
    D. Esophageal intubation

20.67 The most common cause of cardiogenic shock is
    A. Cardiomyopathy
    B. Myocardial contusion from trauma
    C. Acute myocardial infarction (AMI)
    D. Myocarditis

20.68 Which of the following is an absolute contraindication of thrombolytic therapy in AMI?
    A. Previous hemorrhagic stroke
    B. Menses
    C. Defibrillation
    D. Posterior infarction

20.69 Which of the following is **TRUE** regarding DVTs?
    A. They are easily diagnosed by history and physical.
    B. They may be asymptomatic.
    C. A positive Homan sign is both sensitive and specific.
    D. DVTs are not a risk factor for future DVTs.

20.70 Which of the following is considered a risk factor for pulmonary embolism?
    A. Progesterone therapy
    B. Multiparity
    C. History of DVT
    D. Alcoholism

20.71 The initial steps in the treatment of altered mental status of unknown etiology include
    A. Naloxone and D50 IV
    B. Epinephrine 1:1000 SQ and oxygen
    C. Oxygen and stat CT of the head
    D. Blood alcohol level determination

20.72 Which of the following is considered a modifiable risk factor for CVA?
    A. Prior CVA
    B. Family history of CVA
    C. Diabetes mellitus
    D. Age

20.73 According to ACLS guidelines, which of the following is **TRUE** in the evaluation and treatment of CVA?
 A. CT with contrast is used to differentiate hemorrhagic from ischemic stroke.
 B. Thrombolytic therapy should be initiated within 3 to 6 h.
 C. An LP should be performed to rule out a subarachnoid hemorrhage.
 D. tPA and not streptokinase is used for thrombolytic therapy.

20.74 A sudden painless loss of vision in one eye most likely represents
 A. Central retinal artery occlusion
 B. Uveitis
 C. Acute glaucoma
 D. Retinal detachment

20.75 Which of the following physical findings is most consistent with acute angle-closure glaucoma?
 A. Constricted pupil and watery discharge
 B. Normal vision and diffuse injection
 C. Clear cornea and blurred vision
 D. Perilimbal vessel dilation and severe pain

20.76 A patient presents to the ED with a scared, open-mouthed appearance and is unable to talk. Her husband states she yawned and subsequently became very excited, but was unable to tell him why. You suspect
 A. Hyperventilation
 B. Broken tooth
 C. Torticollis
 D. TMJ dislocation

20.77 Initial treatment for the patient in question 20.76 is
 A. Muscle relaxant and reduction of the dislocation
 B. Muscle relaxant and heat to the neck
 C. Immediate referral to a dentist
 D. Rebreathing into a paper bag

20.78 Which of the following statements about cocaine is **TRUE?**
A. It elevates blood pressure and produces bradycardia.
B. It produces tachycardia and increases coronary blood flow.
C. It increases myocardial oxygen consumption and decreases blood pressure.
D. It decreases coronary blood flow and increases myocardial contractility.

20.79 According to BSL guidelines, opening the airway of an unconscious person who has **NOT** suffered trauma should be performed by
A. Head tilt–chin lift
B. Head tilt–neck lift
C. Neck thrust
D. Head tilt–jaw thrust

20.80 According to ACLS guidelines, the first step in the management of asystole is
A. Defibrillation
B. Synchronized cardioversion
C. Confirmation of asystole in two leads
D. Epinephrine 1 mg IV push

Emergency Medicine

Answers and Discussion

20.1 (A) Chest pain and dyspnea are the most common symptoms of spontaneous pneumothorax. (*1, p 471*)

20.2 (D) In a case of tension pneumothorax, you would expect hypotension, marked respiratory distress and cyanosis, deviation of the trachea away from the pneumothorax, and hyperresonance on the side of the pneumothorax. (*1, pp 1613–1616*)

20.3 (C) Performing the other measures prior to chest decompression will assure you of practicing your CPR. (*1, p 471*)

20.4 (D) Expected findings in asthmatic attack include hyperresonance to percussion, prolonged expiratory phase, and expiratory wheezes. Hemoptysis is not an expected finding. (*1, pp 478, 1684*)

20.5 (D) Other causes of wheezing include upper airway obstruction, aspiration of FB, metastatic carcinoma with lymphangitic metastases, sarcoidosis with endobronchial obstruction, and multiple pulmonary emboli. (*1, p 479, Table 64-4*)

20.6 (D) This is the classic presentation of pericarditis. (*1, p 391*)

20.7 (E) Appendicitis is the most common extrauterine surgical emergency in pregnancy. US is useful to exclude adnexal torsion, cholelithiasis, and ectopic pregnancy. (*1, p 537*)

20.8 (C) These are classic symptoms of bowel obstruction. (*1, pp 540–541*)

20.9 (B) Free air indicates perforation, a complication of bowel obstruction. (*1, p 542*)

20.10 (C) This patient is most likely suffering from acute mountain sickness. The most appropriate treatment is oxygen and descent. (*1, pp 1263–1264*)

20.11 (A) Many systems can be involved in decompression sickness, resulting in many symptom possibilities, but hematemesis is not likely. (*1, p 1273*)

20.12 (D) The patient should be placed in a recompression chamber, not necessarily found at the trauma center. If transport is necessary, it should be in a low-flying airplane or in a fully pressurized cabin. Immediate treatment with oxygen and rehydration is advised. (*1, p 1275*)

20.13 (C) This is pulseless V-tach, which is treated as a ventricular fibrillation. (*2, p 41*)

20.14 (B) Other causes of pulseless electrical activity include hypovolemia, tension pneumothorax, and pulmonary embolism. (*2, p 121*)

20.15 (D) The patient is considered unstable; therefore, electrical cardioversion is the most appropriate treatment. (*2, p 135*)

20.16 (A) Cardiovascular side effects are the most common cause of death in tricyclic overdoses. Tricyclics are among the most cardiotoxic medications. (*2, p 111*)

20.17 (A) Patients who do not suffer immediate arrest have an excellent chance of survival; therefore, reverse triage is the rule, with patients in arrest being attended to first. (*2, p 118*)

20.18 (A) The percentage is calculated as follows: trunk, 18%; right arm, 4.5%; right leg, 18%. (*1, p 1282*)

20.19 (B) Tetanus immune status is very important in burn patients, as tetanus immune globulin may be needed in addition to the booster. The other options listed may prove to be deleterious to the patient. (*1, pp 1284–1285*)

20.20 (B) Alternating current causes tetany, thereby inhibiting the victim's release from the source. Most injuries occur to those who work with electricity. (*1, pp 1293–1295*)

20.21 (B) Liquefaction necrosis allows for deeper penetration of the unattached chemical into the tissue. (*1, p 1290*)

20.22 (C) Unless a specific neutralizing agent is readily available, the area that has undergone chemical burns should be immediately and copiously irrigated with water or saline. (*1, p 1287*)

20.23 (B) ECG is appropriate. The others are not indicated. (*1, p 354*)

20.24 (D) Arrhythmias most often account for syncope occurring in seated or lying positions. (*1, pp 352–355*)

20.25 (B) *C. botulinum* can be found in high-risk foods such as home-canned fruits and vegetables, fish and fish products, and condiments. Supportive care and antitoxin are the treatments. (*1, pp 1473–1474*)

20.26 (D) Look for a fine line with hyperlucency and lack of lung markings to indicate pneumothorax. (*1, p 471*)

20.27 (B) Prophylactic antibiotics should be employed because of the location of the bite. (*1, p 335*)

20.28 (B) The history is classic for tetanus. Older patients, especially women, may be nonimmunized or underimmunized, making them a high-risk group. *C. tetani* grows best in the soil of warm, moist climates. (*1, pp 964–967*)

20.29 (D) High-pressure injection injuries to the hand are an emergency best cared for by a hand surgeon. (*1, p 333*)

20.30 (B) CSF analysis is paramount for the diagnosis. (*1, p 1486*)

20.31 (D) In the classic triad of hyperthermia, altered mental status, and seizures, many differential diagnoses must be considered. These include systemic infections, anticholinergic poisoning, thyroid storm, and malignant neuroleptic syndrome. (*1, p 1240*)

20.32 (D) Evaporative cooling is easy, noninvasive, and rapid. The others are effective, but more difficult and/or more invasive. (*1, p 1241*)

20.33 (C) Epinephrine should be the first treatment in cases of potential anaphylactic shock. (*1, pp 1244–1245*)

20.34 (A) The diagnosis of hypothermia can be difficult. Water immersion causes loss of body heat 30 times faster than air. Arrhythmias occur in severe hypothermia or body temperature less than 86°F. (*1, pp 1231–1232*)

20.35 (A) Loss of bladder control is a red flag. This patient should have urgent surgical evaluation. (*1, pp 1252–1253*)

20.36 (C) The envenomated limb should be immobilized. The patient should receive isotonic IV fluids, O_2, and transport to a nearby ER. Cuts and suction should not be attempted. Ice water immersion and tourniquets can only worsen the injury. (*1, pp 1252–1253*)

20.37 (A) In acute compartment syndrome, you would expect excessive pain, numbness, and weakness in the extremity. The affected area may be swollen and tense. Peripheral pulses are often diminished. The acute form usually follows fractures, burns, trauma, or vascular injury. (*1, pp 1868–1869*)

20.38 (D) This patient has superior vena syndrome. All treatments except for diuretics and glucocorticoids are contraindicated. (*1, p 1411*)

20.39 (C) The brown recluse spider is small and rather nondescript, with skinny legs. Paresthesia is not expected. Generalized symptoms may occur, typically 24 to 48 h after the bite. (*1, p 1246*)

20.40 (B) Abdominal rigidity may be mistaken for acute abdomen if the history of spider bite is not obtained. Severe reactions to black widow bite include headache, nausea, bronchorrhea, hypertension, seizures, and altered mental status. Treatment is with analgesics, muscle relaxants, and antivenin. (*1, pp 1247–1248*)

20.41 (B) The site should always be identified in acute epistaxis. (*1, pp 1532–1539*)

20.42 (D) Almost all drowning victims are hypothermic to some extent. (*2, p 11-4*)

20.43 (B) A dose of 140 mg/kg of acetaminophen (less, if the patient has significant underlying liver injury) is hepatotoxic. (*1, p 1126*)

20.44 (D) *N*-acetylcysteine is an effective antidote that prevents hepatotoxicity. Treatment should be started as soon as possible, but is effective if administered within 16 h of ingestion of acetaminophen. (*1, p 1128*)

20.45 (D) The presence of a large number of people in a smoke-filled environment strongly points to carbon monoxide as the most likely cause of their symptoms. (*1, pp 1302–1304*)

20.46 (A) The patient suffering carbon monoxide exposure should be immediately removed from the source of carbon monoxide and given 100% oxygen. (*1, p 1304*)

20.47 (B) Deterioration in the condition of a patient with head injury is a surgical emergency. Loss of consciousness indicates the need for a CT. Head injuries can be masked by drugs or alcohol. (*1, p 1639*)

20.48 (C) Rinse the tooth in tap water, being careful not to handle the root, and replace it in its exact location. (*3, p 219*)

20.49 (A) Any increase in intraocular pressure may expel intraocular contents. A very careful exam and no Valsalva-type maneuvers by the patient are warranted. (*3, p 222*)

20.50 (B) DPL and CT are the most accurate in defining intra-abdominal injury. (*3, p 241*)

20.51 (A) Dissecting abdominal aortic aneurysm is sometimes difficult to diagnose. Look for a pulsatile mass and unequal femoral pulses. All patients over age 50 with these symptoms should be evaluated for AAA. (*3, pp 87–89*)

20.52 (A) Pain is always present in mesenteric ischemia or infarction. The type of pain and other symptoms may vary. (*3, p 89*)

20.53 (A) The symptoms and history and the widened mediastinum should lead immediately to the diagnosis of aortic dissection. The aortogram is the gold standard for diagnosis. (*3, p 93*)

20.54 (D) Testicular torsion typically occurs in the teen years, usually at night, and should be surgically corrected within 6 h. (*3, pp 129–130*)

20.55 (B) Radionuclide scanning is the test of choice for testicular torsion. US is the test of choice for evaluation of a testicular mass. Doppler and UA may aid in the diagnosis. (*3, p 131*)

20.56 (B) Radial pulse requires a systolic blood pressure of at least 80, femoral 70, and carotid 60. (*3, p 196*)

20.57 (E) All are important information in cases of MVA, as are many others. (*3, p 195*)

20.58 (D) Endotracheal intubation is performed in the primary survey, if needed. The other are done in the secondary survey. (*1, p 1611, Table 243-37*)

20.59 (A) Stopping the blood loss is the most effective treatment for hypovolemia secondary to hemorrhage. (*1, p 1610*)

20.60 (B) Cardiac tamponade and tension pneumothorax must be considered. Hypovolemia would not cause flattening of neck veins. Head injury alone has no effect on neck veins. Splenic rupture would result in hypovolemia with flattened neck veins. (*1, p 1159*)

20.61 (D) A human bite to the hand should be left open, not sutured. A hand surgeon should be consulted. (*3, p 255*)

20.62 (A) X-rays do not reveal torn ligaments or meniscal tears. A ruptured patellar tendon requires prompt surgical repair. (*3, p 259*)

20.63 (A) A bucket-handle tear of the meniscus is the most likely cause of locked knee. (*3, p 259*)

20.64 (C) When caring for an amputated part, keep the area moist with a sterile saline dressing. Apply pressure and elevation for bleeding. Splinting helps protect the extremity. (*3, p 264*)

20.65 (A) This is the classic presentation for a peritonsillar abscess. The airway could become compromised; thus consultation with an otolaryngologist is warranted. (*3, p 39*)

20.66 (B) The most common problem is the ET tube being pushed down into the right main stem bronchus. (*2, pp 2–6*)

20.67 (C) All the options listed can cause cardiogenic shock, but AMI is the most common. (*3, p 392*)

20.68 (A) Besides hemorrhagic stroke, absolute contraindications to thrombolytic therapy in AMI include suspected dis secting aortic aneurysm, intracranial neoplasm, and active internal bleeding. (*2, p 1-52*)

20.69 (B) DVTs can be difficult to diagnose and may be asymptomatic. A positive Homan sign is neither sensitive not specific. Having a DVT is a risk factor for future DVTs. (*3, p 425*)

20.70 (C) History of DVT and estrogen treatment are risk factors for pulmonary embolism. (*3, p 469*)

20.71 (A) Steps in treating altered mental status of unknown etiology include drawing blood and giving Narcan, D50, and thiamine. The workup proceeds from there. (*3, p 577*)

20.72 (C) As with MIs, there are many risk factors for CVAs, and many are the same. Modifiable ones include hypertension, cigarette smoking, and diabetes, among others. (*2, p 10-2*)

20.73 (D) CT without contrast is used in evaluating and treating CVA. It must be initiated within 3 h of the onset of symptoms. If subarachnoid hemorrhage is suspected and an LP is performed, thrombolytic therapy cannot be utilized. Streptokinase should not be used in patients with stroke except in clinical studies approved by the Institutional Review Board. (*2, pp 10-2, 10-17*)

20.74 (A) Retinal detachment causes visual field defects such as flashing lights, floaters, or curtain effects. Uveitis and acute glaucoma are both painful. (*3, p 11*)

20.75 (D) Acute angle-closure glaucoma presents with severe pain, nausea/vomiting, and marked decrease in vision. Prompt treatment is necessary to preserve vision. (*3, p 5*)

20.76 (D) In TMJ dislocation, the patient typically presents with a scared, open-mouthed appearance. (*3, p 31; 1, p 1528*)

20.77 (A) Reduction of TMJ dislocation is performed by placing the thumbs on the posterior molars and pushing down and back. (*3, p 31*)

20.78 (D) Cocaine causes elevated blood pressure, tachycardia, increased myocardial contractility, increased myocardial oxygen consumption, and decreased coronary blood flow. (*2, p 11-9*)

20.79 (A) The head tilt–chin lift maneuver is the first maneuver attempted to open the airway of an unconscious person who has not suffered trauma. (*1, p 45*)

20.80 (C) Asystole should not be shocked. It should be confirmed in two leads; the causes should be considered while BLS is initiated. (*2, p 1-23*)

References

1. Tintinalli JE, Kelen GD, Stapczynski JS (eds): *Emergency Medicine: A Comprehensive Study Guide,* 4/e, New York, McGraw-Hill, 1996.

2. Cummins RO (ed): *Textbook of Advanced Cardiac Life Support,* Dallas, American Heart Association, 1997.

3. Harwood-Russ A, Luten RC (eds): *Handbook of Emergency Medicine,* Philadelphia, Lippincott, 1995.

21

Clinical Laboratory Methods

Salah Ayachi, PhD, PA-C

DIRECTIONS (Questions 21.1–21.50): Each of the numbered items or incomplete statements in this chapter is followed by answers or completions of the statement. Select the **one** lettered answer or completion that is **best** in each case.

21.1 A normal pleural tap has
  A. No RBCs
  B. A glucose content of 70 to 100 mg/dL
  C. No WBCs
  D. A protein content of <4.1 g/dL

21.2 Which is **NOT** a sequela of streptococcal pharyngitis?
  A. Hepatomegaly
  B. Cardiomyopathy
  C. Rheumatic fever
  D. Acute glomerulonephritis

21.3 For occult blood in the stool, protocol calls for
  A. Collection of specimens on three consecutive days
  B. Diet counseling to exclude red meats and certain vegetables

    C. Instructions to the patient to return the card to the office or designated laboratory

    D. All of the above

21.4 Which of the following is effective in decontaminating blood and body fluid spills?
    A. Household bleach
    B. Detergent
    C. Scouring cleanser
    D. Copious amounts of water

21.5 The most common anemia, in which hemoglobin and cell sizes are reduced, is due to
    A. Vitamin B_{12} deficiency
    B. Iron deficiency
    C. Folic acid deficiency
    D. Sickle cell disease

21.6 Pregnancy tests may be positive as early as
    A. 2 days after the first missed period
    B. 5 days after conception
    C. 24 h after conception
    D. 7 to 14 days after conception

21.7 A patient presents with symptoms consistent with threatened abortion. She reports that the pregnancy test she took the night before was negative. Which of the following should you consider?
    A. There may be other causes for the patient's symptoms.
    B. The kit she purchased from the local drugstore may yield false results.
    C. The specimen may not have been concentrated enough.
    D. The patient may have used an improper technique.
    E. C and D

21.8 The Kirby-Bauer (disk diffusion) method
    A. Is a test of antibiotic sensitivity
    B. Is best used to test aerobic bacteria that grow rapidly
    C. A and B
    D. None of the above

21.9 Which of the following is correct?
A. Iodide kills *Giardia lamblia,* but chlorine does not.
B. Both iodide and chlorine have bacteriocidal activity.
C. A and B
D. None of the above

21.10 A diagnostic procedure for detecting fungal infections that requires the fungus to be alive by the time it reaches the lab is
A. Wet mount using 10% KOH
B. Skin testing
C. Tissue biopsy
D. Culturing of a lesion

21.11 Which of the following is **NOT** correct concerning the usefulness of sputum cultures?
A. The greater the number of squamous epithelial cells per low-power field, the higher the degree of contamination with oropharyngeal flora.
B. Sputum culture may fail to detect the bacteria responsible for the infection.
C. Some contaminants are potential lower respiratory tract (LRT) pathogens.
D. The presence of large numbers of neutrophils in the sputum more than likely indicates LRT infection.

21.12 Your patient complains of painful, pruritic vesicular lesions on the shaft of his penis. Although you recognize the condition, you order a test to confirm your suspicion. Which test do you order?
A. HSV culture
B. HSV antigen
C. HSV antibody

21.13 Hemolytic disease of the newborn (HDN) is characterized by
A. Maternal and fetal Rh groups that are usually compatible
B. Mild anemia, when present
C. Jaundice due to buildup of unconjugated bilirubin
D. Negative direct Coombs test of infant peripheral blood

21.14 A problem that is associated with the use of stored blood and that produces severe sequelae in patients with liver disease is
A. Loss of RBC vitality leading to spherocytosis
B. Potassium leakage from RBCs
C. Ammonia accumulation
D. Drugs in the blood of donors

21.15 Which of the following statements concerning syphilis is **NOT** correct?
A. The causative agent is *Treponema pallidum.*
B. Antibodies often do not appear until late in the primary stage.
C. Specimen contamination does not affect the results of dark-field examination.
D. Exudate from the ulcer is drawn in a pipette for examination.

21.16 Which is **NOT** a component of the reagent used in current screening tests for syphilis?
A. Cardiolipin
B. Cholesterol
C. Lecithin
D. Bile salts

21.17 In ascertaining pregnancy using urine, the specific gravity of the urine is tested to be sure
A. The urine is not contaminated with proteins
B. The urine is not contaminated with red blood cells
C. The urine is concentrated enough to detect the test hormone
D. The woman is well hydrated prior to collection of the specimen

21.18 Home glucose monitoring is most accurately achieved by
A. Checking urine glucose regularly
B. Determining capillary blood glucose using a glucometer
C. Comparing blood glucose reagent strips to a color chart
D. Performing the test on specimens collected after fasting

21.19 Which is true of hepatitis C and hepatitis C virus (HCV)?
   A. The average incubation period is 6 to 8 wk.
   B. The virus is transmitted in the same manner as hepatitis A virus.
   C. Current lab methods detect the viral antigen halfway during convalescence.
   D. The virus is of the DNA type.

21.20 A patient's blood glucose, determined at a hospital lab, is 170 mg/dL. If the patient uses a home monitor, he or she would expect
   A. Increased blood glucose but normal urine glucose
   B. Increased blood and urine glucose
   C. Normal blood and urine glucose
   D. Normal blood glucose but increased urine glucose

21.21 Cerebrospinal fluid (CSF) is collected to determine central nervous system (CNS) involvement by disease processes. Which is **NOT** true of CSF?
   A. Normally, it is clear or colorless.
   B. CSF glucose level is about 80% that of serum in newborns.
   C. As a general rule, an increased protein concentration roughly correlates with the degree of leucocytosis in the CSF.
   D. Generally, preponderance of polymorphonuclear neutrophils (PMNs) in the CSF indicates viral infections.

21.22 A 10-year-old is brought to your clinic complaining of sore throat. His mother tells you she felt swollen glands in his neck and the boy was feverish. Upon examination, you find the pharynx beefy red with grayish-yellow exudates. Your diagnosis is
   A. Group B β-streptococcus
   B. *Staphylococcus aureus*
   C. *Haemophilus influenzae*
   D. Group A β-streptococcus

21.23 Ferritin, the major iron storage protein, is found in the serum in direct proportion to iron storage. Serum ferritin is elevated in each of the following conditions **EXCEPT**

A. Pregnancy
B. Hemochromatosis
C. Hemolytic anemia
D. Acute inflammation

21.24 Erythrocyte sedimentation rate (ESR) is decreased in
A. Myocardial infarction
B. Pelvic inflammatory disease
C. Rheumatic fever
D. Iron-deficiency anemia

21.25 Cardiac nuclear scanning is used to detect myocardial ischemia, infarction, wall dysmotility, and abnormalities in ejection fraction. What is the main advantage of using ^{99m}Tc sestamibi over ^{201}Tl?
A. The ischemic area is visible several hours after the event.
B. Sestamibi is given orally.
C. Sestamibi is not radioactive.
D. ^{201}Tl is given by the IV route.

21.26 Which of the following conditions does **NOT** produce lymphocytosis?
A. Infectious mononucleosis
B. Viral hepatitis
C. Tuberculosis
D. Use of antineoplastic drugs

21.27 Prostatic acid phosphatase (PAP) levels are decreased in male patients
A. By prostatic manipulation
B. With high alkaline phosphatase
C. With prostate cancer
D. Who are alcoholics

21.28 ACTH stimulation test (a.k.a. cosyntropin test) is used to diagnose adrenal dysfunction using cortisol secretion under exogenous ACTH. With this test, cortisol secretion is exaggerated in
A. Patients with ACTH-producing adrenal tumors
B. Bilateral adrenal hyperplasia
C. Primary adrenal insufficiency
D. Chronic steroid ingestion

21.29 To assess thyroid function using radioactive iodine (^{123}I)
   A. The radioactive material is given by mouth.
   B. The neck is scanned 24 h later.
   C. Areas of abnormal uptake are identified.
   D. A and B
   E. A, B, and C

21.30 Which statement about the small bowel follow-through test is correct?
   A. It is used to identify abnormalities in the large intestine.
   B. Barium transit time is decreased in patients with ileus.
   C. Progression of barium is decreased in patients with malabsorption syndromes.
   D. It is useful in identifying and defining small bowel fistulas.

21.31 Serum gamma-glutamyl transpeptidase (GGT) is
   A. Increased in bone disease
   B. Severalfold higher in newborns than in adults
   C. Decreased by ethanol ingestion
   D. Found in the highest concentrations in skeletal muscle

21.32 In which condition would you expect blood urea nitrogen (BUN) **NOT** to be elevated?
   A. Liver failure
   B. Dehydration
   C. Glomerulonephritis
   D. Starvation

21.33 Glucose-6-phosphate dehydrogenase (G6PD) is involved in the production of NADPH in red blood cells (RBCs). NADPH protects the RBCs from the effects of oxidizing agents. Which of the following ethnic patients are not likely to develop hemolysis when exposed to sulfa drugs?
   A. African Americans
   B. Mexican Americans
   C. Greek Americans
   D. Asian Americans

21.34 The Bethesda System of reporting Pap smear results includes all the following **EXCEPT**

A. Adequacy of the specimen for evaluation
B. Descriptive diagnosis (e.g., cellular, reactive, or infectious changes)
C. Means of collecting the specimen
D. Epithelial cell abnormalities

21.35 Colonoscopy is used to detect pathologic conditions of the rectum, colon, and small bowel. Which of the following disease processes involves concentric layers of the mucosa when viewed with the colonoscope in an adequately prepared bowel?
A. Colon cancer
B. Ulcerative colitis
C. Colon polyps
D. Diverticulosis

21.36 The fibrinogen uptake test using radioactive iodine is used to detect deep venous thrombosis (DVT). Which of the following statements is **TRUE** of this test?
A. It detects only newly formed thrombi or those in the process of forming.
B. Nursing mothers may continue breast-feeding without interruption.
C. False positives may be caused by inflammatory conditions.
D. ^{125}I is not taken up by the thyroid.

21.37 Folic acid levels in the blood are used to evaluate hemolytic disorders and to detect megaloblastic anemia. Which of the following applies to the folic acid test?
A. The patient must fast overnight before the test.
B. Arterial blood, not venous blood, must be used.
C. Folate levels may be decreased by ethanol.
D. Blood may be kept at room temperature for up to 6 h without any effect on the test results.

21.38 Which of the following is a normal cystography finding?
A. Extravasated contrast dye
B. Filling shadows
C. Dye in the ureters
D. Bladder collapse after emptying

21.39 To make a definitive diagnosis of mycobacterial infection (e.g., tuberculosis), sputum is collected, a smear is prepared, and, if indicated, a culture is made. Which is **TRUE** with regard to collection of the specimen?
   A. A single specimen is usually obtained.
   B. The best specimen is collected in the afternoon hours.
   C. The patient may use mouthwash to cleanse the oropharynx prior to collection.
   D. Collection may have to be done by transtracheal aspiration.

21.40 Which of the following factors does **NOT** increase blood glucose?
   A. Stress (e.g., trauma)
   B. Caffeine
   C. Diuretics
   D. Alcohol

21.41 Alveolar (A) to arterial (a) oxygen difference (a.k.a. A-a gradient) is normally less than 10 mm Hg. It is increased in the presence of
   A. Pulmonary edema
   B. Pulmonary fibrosis
   C. Pneumonia
   D. All the above

21.42 Increased aspartate aminotransferase (AST, formerly known as serum glutamic-oxaloacetic transaminase [SGOT]) levels are increased in all the following **EXCEPT**
   A. Hepatitis
   B. Myocardial infarction
   C. Angina pectoris
   D. Alcoholic cirrhosis

21.43 Urinary excretion of uric acid is increased in each of the following **EXCEPT**
   A. Leukemias
   B. High-purine diet
   C. Cancer chemotherapy
   D. Chronic alcoholism

21.44 Which of the diagnostic tests used to visualize the pancreatobiliary system is both diagnostic and therapeutic?
A. Intravenous cholangiography
B. Percutaneous transhepatic cholangiography (PTC)
C. Endoscopic retrograde cholangiopancreatography (ERCP)
D. Oral cholecystography

21.45 Vaccination against hepatitis B is considered successful when
A. HBsAg appears in the serum
B. HBsAb titer is increased in the serum
C. HDV antigen appears in the serum
D. HBsAb disappears from the serum

21.46 Your 28-year-old sexually active female patient complains of a profuse clear vaginal discharge. You suspect
A. Candida species
B. *Chlamydia trachomatis*
C. Bacterial vaginosis
D. Herpes simplex

21.47 A 35-year-old female comes to your clinic complaining of flulike symptoms for the last 2 days. She is concerned because she heard on the news that HIV produces these kinds of symptoms. She also reveals that she has had a "flu shot" about 3 to 4 days earlier. What should you **NOT** tell the patient?
A. In some instances, the vaccine produces a mild case of the flu.
B. The influenza vaccine itself may give a false positive ELISA (screening) test for HIV.
C. She should return to clinic in 5 to 6 wk for an HIV test.
D. The immunoglobulins produced against influenza will protect her against HIV.

21.48 The gold standard for diagnosing maxillary sinusitis is sinus puncture, lavage, and aspiration of secretions from the antrum. Of the other methods in use, which is most cost effective (i.e., provides the best sensitivity and specificity for the money)?
  A. Computed tomography
  B. Magnetic resonance imaging
  C. Standard four-view series radiograph
  D. Single Waters view radiograph

21.49 Pulmonary embolism (PE) remains underdiagnosed and continues to claim the lives of thousands of patients yearly. The gold standard for PE is
  A. CT scan
  B. Ventilation/perfusion (V/Q) scan
  C. Pulmonary angiography
  D. Plasma D-dimer levels

21.50 A 75-year-old man complains of pain with mastication and intermittent diplopia. Which test should you perform initially to help identify the cause of his problems?
  A. Westergren ESR
  B. Temporal artery biopsy
  C. Fundoscopic exam
  D. Refraction error

Clinical Laboratory Methods

Answers and Discussion

21.1 (C) A normal pleural tap should contain no RBCs, but the WBC count can be up to 300 per milliliter. (*1, pp 606–612*)

21.2 (A) There is no indication that the liver is directly affected by streptococcal pharyngitis so as to produce enlargement of that organ. (*2, pp 181–183*)

21.3 (D) A number of factors are known to affect the results of hemoccult testing, including red meats and iron-containing vegetables. Also, clear and appropriate instructions should always be given to the patient. (*2, pp 571–572*)

21.4 (A) Household bleach contains chlorine, which has greater germicidal power than any of the other agents listed. (*2, p 220*)

21.5 (B) The most common cause of anemia, especially in the pediatric and geriatric populations, is insufficient intake of iron. In adolescents and adults with severe enough deficiency to produce anemia, bleeding is the most common cause. Furthermore, cell size (MCV) is decreased in approximately 65% of cases of chronic iron deficiency. (*2, pp 11, 22, 25*)

21.6 (D) Many different pregnancy test kits are available on the market. Most tests are based on immunoassays that detect β-human chorionic gonadotropin (β-hCG) in either serum or urine. These tests can detect this hormone as early as 1 to 2 wk after conception. (*2, p 544*)

21.7 (E) The two factors that have an impact on pregnancy testing outcome are the specimen concentration and the technique used. A specimen that is not concentrated enough will more than likely give a false negative result. Similarly, improper technique gives erroneous results. (*2, p 544*)

21.8 (C) The Kirby-Bauer (K-B) method is the most commonly used method of determining the sensitivity of bacteria to different classes of antibiotics. After appropriate steps in the preparation of bacterial culture, a plate that has disks impregnated with representative antibiotics is streaked with the bacteria. Following incubation, the plate is observed for clear areas around each of the disks, which represent inhibition of bacterial growth. (*2, p 222*)

21.9 (C) Whereas both iodide and chlorine kill bacteria, only iodide kills *G. lamblia,* a parasitic agent that causes diarrhea. (*2, p 222*)

21.10 (D) A fungal agent must be alive to be cultured. (*2, pp 237–238*)

21.11 (D) The presence of large numbers of segmented neutrophils in sputum cultures may be due to either upper or lower respiratory tract infection. (*2, p 214*)

21.12 (A) The gold standard for detecting the presence of herpes simplex virus is the culture. (*1, p 657*)

21.13 (C) Destruction of fetal RBCs by maternal antibodies causes bilirubin to accumulate, leading to jaundice. Incompatibility, which most often resides in the Rh groups, leads to variable degrees of anemia (in some cases fatal). The direct Coombs test is positive in these cases. (*2, pp 135–137*)

21.14 (C) Spherocytosis may cause confusion as to whether the donor may have an autoimmune disease. RBCs in stored blood lose vitality and undergo membrane changes that allow escape of potassium; this would most affect recipients with renal disease. Drugs in donor blood would affect any recipient if found in sufficient quantities. However, ammonia, levels of which can rise severalfold in old blood, would be most detrimental to a recipient with severe liver disease. (*2, p 144*)

21.15 (C) Red blood cells obscure the spirochetes and interfere with dark-field examination. (*2, p 226*)

21.16 (D) Bile salts are not a component of the lipoprotein mixture to which antibodies are produced. (*2, p 227*)

21.17 (C) Several factors have to be considered when testing for human chorionic gonadotropin (hCG) in the urine; the assays determine the concentration of this hormone in the urine. Therefore, the extent to which urine is concentrated or diluted will affect the results. Specific gravity is a simple way to determine urine concentration. (*2, p 544*)

21.18 (B) Glucosuria develops only when the kidneys' reabsorptive capacity is surpassed. With fasting, blood glucose levels may fall below the threshold and no glucose will appear in the urine. Comparison of reagent strips to a color chart is subjective and depends on the patient's visual acuity and ability to distinguish colors. Therefore, presuming proper collection technique and timing, the glucometer will give the most accurate results. (*2, pp 151–153*)

21.19 (A) HCV is an RNA virus that is transmitted much in the manner of hepatitis B virus. Its incubation period lasts 6 to 8 wk. Currently, serologic tests are aimed at detecting the antibody to HCV. Although the antigen can be detected 2 to 4 wk after infection, when nucleic acid probes are used, it becomes nondetectable at the beginning of convalescence. (*2, pp 257–259*)

21.20 (A) Urine glucose will be normal because the renal threshold (180 mg/dL) is not surpassed, and all filtered glucose is reabsorbed; therefore, none should spill into the urine. (*2, p 150*)

21.21 (D) As a general rule, bacterial involvement of the CNS causes increases in PMNs. (*2, pp 294–296*)

21.22 (D) Streptococcal pharyngitis is most prevalent in children up to age 13. This is a case where a rapid strep test is warranted in order to commence therapy with a suitable antibiotic as soon as possible to avoid complications. (*2, pp 181–183*)

21.23 (A) Anemia is very common in pregnancy because of disproportionate increases in plasma volume (50%) vs. red cell volume (25%), and because women often suffer from iron-deficiency anemia. With the decrease in iron, there is proportionate decrease in serum ferritin levels. (*3, p 770*)

21.24 (D) ESR is a nonspecific test that is affected by many disease processes. It is expressed in millimeters per hour. It is increased with injury (e.g., myocardial infarction), inflammation, infections, and diseases associated with increased serum proteins. ESR is decreased in severe iron-deficiency anemia. (*1, pp 199–201*)

21.25 (A) ^{201}Tl is picked up by normal cells, leaving ischemic areas "cold," whereas sestamibi highlights ischemic cells for hours after the ischemic event. (*1, pp 704–705*)

21.26 (D) Antineoplastic drugs decrease white blood cell production. (*1, p 867*)

21.27 (D) Alcohol and several other drugs (e.g., heparin) lower PAP levels, whereas manipulation of the prostate, as during a rectal exam, increases PAP. In prostate cancer, PAP levels are used to monitor the disease process. (*1, pp 20–22*)

21.28 (B) Cortisol secretion is exaggerated with ACTH administration when the condition is due to bilateral adrenal hyperplasia, but not with primary dysfunction of adrenal suppression by chronic steroid intake. (*1, pp 26–28*)

21.29 (E) To assess thyroid function, radioactive iodine is given to the patient, provided he or she is not allergic to iodine. Twenty-four hours later, a detector is passed over the patient's neck, and uptake is recorded. Uptake characteristics are used to determine the degree of activity of glandular tissue as well as its anatomic features. (*1, pp 740–743*)

21.30 (D) For small bowel follow-through, the patient either swallows the barium or is given the material by nasogastric tube if he or she cannot swallow. Serial x-rays, taken at specific time intervals, are used to assess progression of the barium through the small intestine. In the case of ileus (decreased motility), transit time is increased; in malabsorption syndromes, however, the barium transit time is shortened. Fistulas, obstructions, and tumors can be identified by this technique. (*1, pp 990–993*)

21.31 (B) Although children have GGT levels similar to those of adults, newborns have about five times as much GGT. Organs that contain the highest GGT levels are the liver, kidneys, spleen, and prostate. GGT determination is useful in the evaluation of alcoholics and in patients with hepatic damage. (*1, pp 219–221*)

21.32 (A) BUN is made in the liver and excreted by the kidneys. While liver failure decreases BUN production, renal disease leads to decreased excretion of this metabolic product. Starvation increases it because of increased protein catabolism. (*1, pp 443–446*)

21.33 (D) Of the ethnic groups listed, only Mexican Americans are not at risk of the genetic defect of glucose 6-phosphate dehydrogenase (G6PD) deficiency. African Americans have the highest risk. (*1, pp 231–233*)

21.34 (C) How the Pap smear specimen is collected and prepared is not part of the report submitted by the pathologist. However, whether or not the specimen is adequate for interpretation is a determination made by the reader. (*1, pp 666–670*)

21.35 (A) Of the conditions listed, colon cancer involves concentric layers of mucosa. All others are more limited in extent. (*1, pp 522–526*)

21.36 (C) Areas of inflammation within the suspected limb may take up radiolabeled fibrinogen, thereby giving false positive results. (*1, pp 709–711*)

21.37 (C) The patient having folic acid levels tested should refrain from imbibing alcohol if reliable results are to be obtained. Ethanol is one of several drugs known to decrease folate levels. (*1, pp 217–219*)

21.38 (D) Filling shadows (defects) usually indicate primary tumors in the bladder, while the presence of dye outside it indicates traumatic rupture or perforation. The presence of dye in the ureters usually indicates reflux of urine from the bladder into the ureters (vesicoureteral reflux). (*1, pp 948–950*)

21.39 (D) Usually three separate sputum specimens are obtained, if necessary by means other than coughing (e.g., transtracheal aspiration, bronchoscopy, etc.). The patient should be instructed not to use mouthwash, but encouraged to rinse out any food particles and saliva with water. The best specimens are those obtained after the patient awakens. (*1, pp 636–638*)

21.40 (D) Many factors increase serum glucose, just as many others decrease it. Of the items listed, only alcohol decreases serum glucose. (*1, pp 233–238*)

21.41 (E) All the conditions listed are known to increase respiratory membrane thickness and hinder the exchange of oxygen between alveoli and vasculature. Other conditions that lead to mixing of deoxygenated blood (e.g., septal defects and others) also increase the A a gradient. (*1, p 100*)

21.42 (C) AST is released in the bloodstream following cell injury in the heart or liver. However, in angina there is ische mia but no cell disruption, and consequently no enzyme release. (*1, p 106*)

21.43 (D) Chronic ethanol ingestion decreases renal tubular excretion of uric acid because of the chronic acidosis associated with chronic ethanolism. (*1, pp 858–859*)

21.44 (C) ERCP is used to visualize the pancreas and bile ducts, but can also be used to decompress the pancreatobiliary system. It is difficult to perform, thus the complications that ensue. PTC allows visualization and decompression of the biliary system. It too is difficult to perform and is fraught with complications. (*1, pp 532–536*)

21.45 (B) Vaccination is successful when the antibody to hepatitis B virus can be recovered in the serum. HDV antigen signifies a coinfection. (*1, pp 260–263*)

21.46 (A) Infections of vaginal origin include candida species, bacterial vaginosis, and *Trichomonas vaginalis*. (*4, p 256*)

21.47 (D) It is well established that recent vaccination against influenza can produce false positive HIV tests. Since the patient appears apprehensive about the possibility of being HIV positive, you would do well to recognize that, explain the effect of the vaccine, and recommend she return to clinic later for HIV testing. (*4, p 273*)

21.48 (D) Single Waters view radiographs have been reported to provide specificity that is higher than that of MRI and nearly the same as that provided by four-view radiography. (*4, p 298*)

21.49 (C) Pulmonary angiography, which carries serious risks because of its invasive nature, remains the gold standard for the diagnosis of PE. A new method that is receiving much attention calls for determining the levels of plasma D-dimers, which are products of fibrinolysis, as markers of PE. (*4, pp 330–332*)

21.50 (A) The main concern in this patient is the possibility that temporal (giant cell) arteritis (TA) is the cause of his symptoms. Because of the need for therapy to avoid morbidity, the ESR should be performed. If it is elevated, a biopsy of the temporal artery should be considered. (*4, p 433*)

References

1. Pagana KD, Pagana TJ: *Mosby's Manual of Diagnostic and Laboratory Tests,* St. Louis, Mosby, 1998.

2. Ravel R: *Clinical Laboratory Medicine—Clinical Application of Laboratory Data,* 6/e, St. Louis, Mosby, 1995.

3. Crombelholme WR: Obstetrics. In: Tierney LM, McPhee SJ, Papadakis MA (eds): *Current Medical Diagnosis & Treatment,* New York, McGraw-Hill, 2000.

4. Black ER, Bordley DR, Tape TG, et al (eds): *Diagnostic Strategies for Common Medical Problems,* Philadelphia, American College of Physicians, 1999.

22

Pharmacology

Salah Ayachi, PhD, PA-C

DIRECTIONS (Questions 22.1–22.80): Each of the numbered items or incomplete statements in this chapter is followed by answers or completions of the statement. Select the **one** lettered answer or completion that is **best** in each case.

22.1 Potassium-sparing diuretics
- **A.** Cause more sodium excretion than do thiazides
- **B.** Are effective antihypertensives when given alone
- **C.** Should not be used concurrently with salt substitutes
- **D.** Produce hypokalemia when given together with ACE inhibitors

22.2 Which is **NOT** a contraindication to ACE inhibitor therapy?
- **A.** Symptomatic hypotension
- **B.** Renal insufficiency
- **C.** Hyperkalemia that cannot be ameliorated
- **D.** Intolerance to ACE inhibitors
- **E.** History of congestive heart failure

22.3 Endocarditis prophylaxis is recommended in
- **A.** Tympanostomy tube insertion
- **B.** Cesarean section
- **C.** Dental procedures not likely to produce gingival bleeding
- **D.** Prostatic surgery

22.4 Treatment of peptic ulcer disease (PUD) should take into consideration that
   A. Ulcer recurrence may be as high as 80% within 12 mo
   B. "Triple therapy" reduces the recurrence rate to 5% or less
   C. Only 10% to 20% of those infected with *Helicobacter pylori* develop PUD
   D. All of the above

22.5 *H. pylori* has been implicated in
   A. Peptic ulcer disease
   B. Gastric ulcer disease
   C. Chronic active gastritis
   D. A and B
   E. A, B, and C

22.6 Rational and effective treatment of mycobacterial tuberculosis (MTB) is predicated on all of the following **EXCEPT**
   A. Early diagnosis
   B. Use of a single anti-TB agent
   C. Selection of the proper therapeutic regimen
   D. Maintaining a high degree of suspicion for noncompliance

22.7 Which of the following is a prophylactic agent for *Pneumocystis carinii* pneumonia (PCP)?
   A. Trimethoprim-sulfamethoxazole (Bactrim)
   B. Dapsone
   C. Pentamidine
   D. Fluconazole (Diflucan)
   E. A, B, and C

22.8 The antidepressant associated with the highest incidence of orthostatic hypotension is
   A. Amitriptyline (Elavil)
   B. Sertraline (Zoloft)
   C. Fluoxetine (Prozac)
   D. Trazodone (Desyrel)

22.9 Your patient has a pseudomonas infection. Which of the following is indicated for treatment?
A. Cephalexin (Keflex)
B. Cefuroxime (Ceftin)
C. Cefaclor (Ceclor)
D. Ceftazidime (Fortaz)

22.10 One year ago, your patient had to be hospitalized for a reaction to penicillin. He now has community-acquired pneumonia that is sensitive to penicillin. What drug would you give him?
A. Augmentin
B. Cefixime
C. Ciprofloxacin
D. Cephalexin

22.11 Cortisporin otic suspensions are contraindicated in patients with
A. Perforated eardrum
B. Fungal infection
C. Ear discharge
D. Asthma

22.12 Your patient has chronic renal insufficiency. The results of the 24-h urine collection you ordered show a creatinine clearance of 20 cc/min. Which diuretic should you prescribe for this patient?
A. Triamterene (Dyrenium)
B. Hydrochlorothiazide (Hydrodiuril)
C. Furosemide (Lasix)
D. Spironolactone (Aldactone)

22.13 Which of the following is **NOT** managed with dexamethasone?
A. Allergic conditions
B. Collagen diseases
C. Cerebral edema
D. Cushing syndrome

22.14 Your patient has a pseudomonas infection that you decide to treat with ciprofloxacin. Your patient also has GERD. Which of the following would be most useful in the treatment of GERD?
A. Sucralfate (Carafate)
B. Ranitidine (Zantac)
C. Tums
D. Milk of magnesia

22.15 Digoxin (Lanoxin) dosing should be reduced in patients with
A. Liver disease
B. Renal dysfunction
C. Congestive heart failure
D. Paroxysmal atrial tachycardia

22.16 H_2 receptor blockers such as cimetidine and ranitidine
A. Are cytoprotective
B. Are more effective than proton pump inhibitors
C. Decrease acid production in the stomach
D. Increase lower esophageal sphincter tone

22.17 You explain to your patient that he should not exceed the prescribed dose of furosemide (Lasix). When brought in to the clinic by his granddaughter, he is dehydrated. You order lytes and ABGs as part of your workup. What would you expect to find?
A. Hyperkalemia and alkalosis
B. Hypochloremia and acidosis
C. Hypokalemia and acidosis
D. Hypokalemia and alkalosis

22.18 Which of the following statements regarding enoxaparin is **INCORRECT?**
A. It is a low-molecular-weight heparin fraction.
B. It produces its anticoagulant effect by binding to antithrombin.
C. It inhibits vitamin K synthesis.
D. It is indicated for primary prevention of deep venous thrombosis.

22.19 Which of the following is a first-line antibiotic in the treatment of *Bordetella pertussis?*
  A. Trimethoprim/sulfamethoxazole
  B. Tetracycline
  C. Amoxicillin
  D. Erythromycin

22.20 Vitamin E consists of a group of naturally occurring fat-soluble nutrients known as tocopherols. Which of the following effect(s) has been attributed to vitamin E?
  A. It improves walking distance and blood flow in patients with intermittent claudication.
  B. It reduces the risk of radiation- and chemical-induced cancers.
  C. In conjunction with zidovudine (AZT), it enhances immune system resistance to opportunistic infections associated with AIDS.
  D. A and B
  E. A, B, and C

22.21 Which of the following antihypertensive agents is centrally acting?
  A. Enalapril (Vasotec)
  B. Metolazone (Zaroxolyn)
  C. Digoxin (Lanoxin)
  D. Clonidine (Catapres)

22.22 Which of the following antibiotics interferes with bacterial DNA replication?
  A. Tircacillin
  B. Erythromycin
  C. Vancomycin
  D. Ciprofloxacin

22.23 Which of the following medications is **NOT** ototoxic?
  A. Hydrochlorothiazide
  B. Gentamicin
  C. Streptomycin
  D. Furosemide

22.24 Which of the following increases the risk of aminoglycoside ototoxicity?
A. Impaired renal function
B. Impaired hepatic function
C. Previous exposure to aminoglycosides
D. Any of the above

22.25 Clindamycin (Cleocin) is a protein-synthesis-inhibiting antibiotic. It is a first-choice antibiotic in the treatment of
A. Gram-positive cocci
B. *Staphylococcus aureus*
C. *Toxoplasma gondii*
D. Mixed anaerobic-aerobic intraabdominal and pelvic infections

22.26 Tetracyclines are indicated for all of the following **EXCEPT**
A. Rickettsiae
B. Lyme disease
C. Mycoplasma
D. *S. aureus*

22.27 The apparent volume of distribution (aVd) of a drug, calculated by dividing its total amount in the body by its plasma concentration, differs with various drugs. Which statement is correct?
A. Some drugs have aVd in excess of the total volume of the body.
B. Lipid-soluble drugs have a high aVd.
C. Drugs that are avidly bound to plasma proteins have a low aVd.
D. A and B
E. A, B, and C

22.28 Your 48-year-old patient with a seizure disorder treated with phenytoin (Dilantin) has recently been found to have multidrug-resistant tuberculosis. You decide to use an antitubercular regimen that includes rifampin and isoniazid (INH). Which of the following is correct?
   A. The same Dilantin dose will be indicated.
   B. Serum Dilantin levels will be increased by rifampin.
   C. The antitubercular regimen will be inadequate.
   D. The patient may experience breakthrough seizures.

22.29 Which of the following is used to treat toxoplasmosis?
   A. Bactrim
   B. Albendazole
   C. Pyrimethamine
   D. Pentamidine

22.30 Which of the following is **NOT** true of INH?
   A. It is used together with other agents for the treatment of tuberculosis.
   B. It is effective against other mycobacteria (e.g., *Mycobacterium kansasii, Mycobacterium marinum*).
   C. It is used in conjunction with vitamin B_6 to reduce the incidence of neuropathy.
   D. It is more rapidly metabolized in Asians than in Caucasians.

22.31 Your patient is HIV positive with CD4 = 335 and viral load (VL) = 48,000. He has recurrent furunculosis originally determined to be due to *S. aureus*. You decide to add another agent to the cephalosporin you started him on. Which antibiotic should you consider?
   A. Doxycycline
   B. Rifampin
   C. Chloramphenicol
   D. Metronidazole

22.32 Which of the following serum changes do you **NOT** expect in a patient treated with spironolactone (Aldactone)?
   A. Hypercalcemia
   B. Hyperkalemia
   C. Acidosis
   D. Hypomagnesemia

22.33 Kinins have been found to exert differential effects on blood vessels. Which is true of kinins?
A. They are involved in maintaining ductus arteriosus patency.
B. They dilate large arteries and veins.
C. They dilate small arteries (arterioles).
D. They dilate umbilical vessels.

22.34 Antineoplastic drugs have different modes of action. Which of the following acts by cross-linking DNA strands?
A. Vinblastine
B. Methotrexate
C. Cyclophosphamide
D. Bleomycin

22.35 Histamine is a powerful chemical that acts on many different tissues through three types of receptors. Which of these receptors is self-regulatory (i.e., when activated, leads to inhibition of release of histamine and other transmitters whose release is mediated by histamine)?
A. H_1
B. H_2
C. H_3
D. A and B

22.36 Angiotensin II receptor blocking agents such as Losartan exert a direct inhibitory effect on the secretion of
A. Renin
B. Aldosterone
C. Antidiuretic hormone (ADH)
D. None of the above

22.37 Which of the following can be used for empiric therapy for bacterial pneumonia in a 45-year-old man whom you see in the emergency department?
A. Levofloxacin
B. Erythromycin
C. Amoxicillin/clavulanate
D. A or B
E. A, B, or C

22.38 Which of the following causes adverse drug reactions in the elderly?
A. Prescription of a high-risk drug to a vulnerable patient
B. Prescription of a highly interactive drug to a vulnerable patient
C. Automatic drug prescribing (as in standard orders in CCUs)
D. Failure to adjust dosages
E. Any of the above

22.39 Nonsteroidal anti-inflammatory drugs (NSAIDs) are among the most important causes of morbidity and mortality in the elderly. Which of the following adverse reactions are associated with these drugs?
A. Gastritis
B. Peptic ulceration
C. Renal insufficiency
D. A and B
E. A, B, and C

22.40 Which is **NOT** a likely sequela of long-term estrogen therapy?
A. Carbohydrate intolerance
B. Thromboembolic events
C. Osteopenia
D. Menstrual changes

22.41 Isotretinoin (Acutane) is restricted to treatment of severe cystic acne. Although effective, it has several side effects, including
A. Dryness of skin and mucous membranes
B. Excessive hair growth
C. Increased appetite
D. Short half-life of 4 to 6 h

22.42 Ionized substances, including antibiotics, do not cross the blood-brain barrier (BBB). In meningitis, such substances gain access to the brain because
A. Inflamed meninges are more permeable.
B. Ionized substances become nonpolar.

   C. Ionized substances increase capillary hydrostatic pressure.
   D. Nonpolar substances penetrate the BBB.

22.43 Pelvic inflammatory disease (PID) is a major cause of infertility but, in many cases, is clinically silent. For best compliance and given the adverse effects of these drugs, which of the following treatment regimens would you institute?
   A. Zithromax 500 mg IV followed by 250 mg PO × 6 days
   B. Zithromax in combination with metronidazole
   C. Metronidazole 500 mg IV bid followed by 500 mg PO × 11 days
   D. Any of the above

22.44 Phase IV of drug testing in humans refers to
   A. Defining the range of doses tolerated by human volunteers
   B. Initial controlled trials to show efficacy
   C. Extensive multicenter trials to corroborate data from earlier results
   D. Research after the drug is marketed to uncover new indications and/or rare adverse effects

22.45 Which of the following antiviral regimens can be used to treat genital herpes?
   A. Acyclovir 400 mg PO tid for 7 to 10 days for first episodes
   B. Valcyclovir 500 mg PO bid for 5 days for episodic flare-ups
   C. Famciclovir 250 mg PO bid for daily suppressive therapy
   D. Acyclovir 5 to 10 mg/kg IV every 8 h for 5 to 7 days for severe disease
   E. Any of the above

22.46 The absorption and bioavailability of a drug are important parameters, but do not indicate how effective the drug is. Another parameter (distribution) depends on
  A. Drug solubility
  B. Anatomic barriers
  C. Organ size and blood flow to that organ
  D. All of the above

22.47 Biotransformations of drugs fall into two phases. Which of the following is a phase II type of reaction?
  A. Hydroxylation
  B. Methylation
  C. Hydrolysis
  D. Oxide formation

22.48 A smoker has decided to heed your admonition regarding harmful effects of smoking and to quit smoking cigarettes. The proper way to treat this patient is to
  A. Encourage him or her to substitute cigars for cigarettes
  B. Ask him or her to chew nicotine-containing gum
  C. Provide him or her with a transdermal source of decreasing nicotine levels
  D. Have him or her stop cold turkey

22.49 If a drug is eliminated from the body according to the zero-order model (i.e., elimination rate is constant regardless of concentration), and its half-life is 20 h, how many hours would it take to eliminate 87.5% of a single dose of the drug?
  A. 30
  B. 40
  C. 80
  D. 60

22.50 Ergot alkaloids have been used to treat acute attacks of migraine headaches. Since their effect is, at least partly, through α-adrenergic agonism, these drugs are contraindicated in
  A. Cases of bradycardia
  B. Patients with coronary artery disease

C. Individuals with moderate to severe hypertension
D. A and B
E. A, B, and C

22.51 Increased serum levels of prolactin are associated with anterior pituitary tumors. In both males and females, this condition results in galactorrhea. Which of the following ergot alkaloids can be used to suppress the tumors and control the galactorrhea (even though no longer indicated for it per the FDA as of 1995)?
A. Ergonovine
B. Ergotamine
C. LSD
D. Bromocriptine

22.52 When a drug loses its effectiveness in a patient who has been treated with it, the patient is said to have developed
A. Tachyphylaxis
B. Hypersensitivity
C. Hyperreactivity
D. Desensitization

22.53 A number of antihypertensive drugs produce orthostatic hypotension as a side effect. One such drug is prazosin (Minipress), which is an α_1 blocker used to control essential hypertension. Prazosin and its newer analogs also
A. Decrease low-density lipoproteins in the serum
B. Are used to treat benign prostatic hypertrophy
C. Are used to treat congestive heart failure
D. A and C

22.54 The effective concentration of digoxin in blood is >0.8 ng/ml and the toxic concentration is >2 ng/ml. This means digoxin
A. Has a narrow therapeutic index
B. Has a long half-life
C. Is lipophilic
D. Blocks the Na^+, K^+ adenosine triphosphatase
E. B, C, and D

22.55 Hypertensive emergencies lead to cerebrovascular hemorrhage, left ventricular failure, or myocardial infarction. Therefore it is imperative that treatment be instituted as soon as possible. Which of the following is the most rapidly acting drug used in hypertensive emergencies?
  A. Hydralazine
  B. Nitroprusside
  C. Labetolol
  D. Clonidine

22.56 Chronic corticosteroid therapy has a number of adverse effects that include
  A. Glucose intolerance
  B. Myopathy
  C. Cataracts
  D. A and B
  E. A, B, and C

22.57 A slow infusion of norepinephrine (NE) in a heart transplant patient will
  A. Increase blood pressure
  B. Increase myocardial contractility
  C. Produce reflex bradycardia
  D. A and B

22.58 Which of the following receptor–blocking agent pairs is **NOT** properly matched?
  A. Beta receptors—propranolol (Inderal)
  B. Muscarinic receptors—atropine
  C. α_1 receptors—phentolamine
  D. α_2 receptors—tyramine

22.59 Infective endocarditis may occur following dental surgery and affect rheumatic or congenitally abnormal valves. Which can be used to treat oral infections in a penicillin-allergic patient?
  A. Penicillin G
  B. Doxycycline
  C. Erythromycin
  D. Ciprofloxacin

22.60 Which of these drugs should **NOT** be stopped preoperatively?
  A. Oral hypoglycemics
  B. Diuretics
  C. Warfarin
  D. Antibiotics

22.61 Dopamine (Intropin) may be used in severe shock to
  A. Increase arterial pressure
  B. Improve perfusion of peripheral tissues
  C. Dilate renal blood vessels
  D. A and B
  E. A, B, and C

22.62 Sildenafil (Viagra) is a potent vasodilator that
  A. Increases blood flow into the penis
  B. Is well tolerated by men with good exercise tolerance
  C. Has resulted in the deaths of patients treated with nitrates
  D. A and B
  E. A, B, and C

22.63 Patients with a history of bronchospasms, diabetes, or peripheral vascular disease who require beta blockers would benefit from
  A. Atenolol (Tenormin)
  B. Pindolol (Visken)
  C. Metoprolol (Lopressor)
  D. A and C

22.64 Identify the correct match of drug(s) and treatment objective in angina management.
  A. Aspirin—reduce preload
  B. Nitrates—reduce oxygen demand
  C. Calcium channel blockers—decrease vascular compliance
  D. Beta blockers—reduce preload

22.65 Thiazide diuretics have been in use for treatment of hypertension for many years. Recently, they have been linked to cardiac sudden deaths when given in high doses. Given the mechanism of action of thiazides, what is the most likely reason for these deaths?
A. Congestive heart failure
B. Hyperkalemia
C. Hypomagnesemia
D. Hypocalcemia

22.66 The optimum duration of therapy for uncomplicated cystitis is 7 days for patients
A. With diabetes mellitus
B. With more than 7 days of symptoms
C. Who are pregnant
D. A and B
E. A, B, and C

22.67 Generally, black patients do not respond as well as do nonblacks to the following antihypertensive drug(s)
A. Beta blockers
B. ACE inhibitors
C. Calcium channel blockers
D. A and B

22.68 Which one of the following is known to interfere with calcium reabsorption by the renal tubules and, therefore, can be used to treat hypercalcemia?
A. Hydrochlorothiazide
B. Nifedipine
C. Digoxin
D. Furosemide

22.69 Which of the following calcium channel blocker(s) is useful in managing supraventricular tachycardia and reducing ventricular response in atrial fibrillation?
A. Nifedipine
B. Verapamil
C. Diltiazem
D. B and C
E. A, B, and D

22.70 Your patient is hypertensive and suffers from bouts of depression treated with amitriptyline (Elavil). If you opt to treat the patient with a calcium channel blocker, which would you avoid because of constipating action?
A. Verapamil
B. Diltiazem
C. Nifedipine
D. Felodipine

22.71 Which of the following drugs is **NOT** a central nervous system (CNS) stimulant?
A. Cocaine
B. Nicotine
C. Caffeine
D. Methadone

22.72 Selective serotonin reuptake inhibitors (SSRIs) such as Prozac are more desirable than tricyclic antidepressants (TCAs) because SSRIs
A. Have no anticholinergic activity
B. Are not toxic in overdose
C. Lack cardiotoxic adverse effects
D. A and B
E. A, B, and C

22.73 Which of the following is an HIV protease inhibitor?
A. Didanosine (Videx, DDI)
B. Stavudine (Zerit, D4T)
C. Lamivudine (Epivir, 3TC)
D. Nelfinavir (Viracept)

22.74 Prophylactic treatment of migraine headaches is designed to reduce their frequency, duration, and intensity. One agent that has been used to treat insomnia and has proven useful in migraine prophylaxis is
A. Amitriptyline
B. Propranolol
C. Verapamil
D. Ergotamine

22.75 Of the antifungal agents listed, which affects host cells as well as fungal cells?
A. Clotrimazole
B. Fluconazole
C. Amphotericin B
D. Itraconazole

22.76 Which of the following antiviral drugs is well known for its adverse effects of peripheral neuropathy and pancreatitis?
A. Zidovudine
B. Nelfinavir
C. Acyclovir
D. Didanosine

22.77 Antiviral agents used to treat cytomegalovirus (CMV) infections in AIDS patients include
A. Ganciclovir
B. Foscarnet
C. Acyclovir
D. A and B

22.78 Human immunodeficiency virus (HIV) is an RNA virus. Saquinavir (Fortovase, Invirase) is used to halt replication of this virus by interfering with
A. Viral adsorption
B. Reverse transcriptase activity
C. Assembly and release of new viruses
D. All of the above

22.79 Glipizide, a second-generation sulfonylurea, interacts with several drugs. Which of the following is a correct match of glipizide-drug interaction?
A. Alcohol—disulfiram-like reaction
B. Thiazides—hypoglycemia
C. Cimetidine—hyperglycemia
D. Warfarin—hyperglycemia

22.80 A chronic alcoholic patient complains of abdominal pain and foul-smelling, clay-colored stools. What medication would be appropriate for his condition?

A. Metronidazole (Flagyl)

B. Loperamide (Imodium)

C. Ibuprofen (Motrin)

D. Pancreolipase preparation

Pharmacology

Answers and Discussion

22.1 (C) Potassium-sparing diuretics should not be given with salt substitutes, which are K^+ salts. They should not be administered with ACE inhibitors because they have additive hyperkalemic effects. (*1, p 221*)

22.2 (E) ACE inhibitors have been found effective in the treatment of congestive heart failure. Compared to other agents, they have few side effects, other than hypotension. (*1, p 177*)

22.3 (D) Prostatic surgery is likely to cause transient bacteremia involving enterococci, one of the two agents involved in nearly 60% of cases of infectious endocarditis (the others being streptococci). (*1, p 404*)

22.4 (D) All three statements are true. (*1, p 306*)

22.5 (E) Patients with peptic and gastric ulcer disease have been found to harbor *H. pylori;* chronic active gastritis is also linked to the same agent. (*1, p 306*)

22.6 (B) A single agent is no longer an appropriate therapeutic choice for MTB given the incidence of drug resistance and other factors, including noncompliance. (*2, p 03*)

22.7 (E) Fluconazole is an antifungal agent. Bactrim is the drug of choice for prophylactic treatment of PCP. Individuals with hypersensitivity to sulfa drugs may be treated with daily doses of dapsone or a monthly dose of aerosolized pentamidine. (*3, p 740*)

22.8 (A) The hypotensive effect of amitriptyline is due to its α_1 receptor antagonism. (*4, p 291*)

22.9 (D) Ceftazidime is a third-generation cephalosporin more effective than any of those listed with respect to coverage of both *Pseudomonas aeruginosa* and *S. aureus.* (*5, p 711*)

22.10 (D) A first-generation cephalosporin may be used cautiously to treat community-acquired pneumonia in patients without COPD who are known to be penicillin allergic, even though cross-sensitivity with cephalosporins is estimated at 10%. This is to reduce the cost associated with using broad-spectrum antibiotics (such as ciprofloxacin) and the incidence of resistance development. (*6, pp 245–246*)

22.11 (B) Cortisporin contains hydrocortisone (HC), polymyxin B sulfate, and neomycin, none of which has any antifungal activity. In fact, HC favors fungal growth because of its immunosuppressant effects. (*7, p 81*)

22.12 (C) Furosemide and other high-ceiling diuretics are used in patients who do not respond to thiazides, namely those with decreased renal function (e.g., decreased GFR and elevated serum creatinine or blood urea nitrogen [BUN]). (*8, p 157*)

22.13 (A) Dexamethasone (Decadron) is used to treat each of the conditions listed except Cushing syndrome. In Cushing syndrome it is used in the "overnight suppression test" to diagnose the condition. (*9, p 145*)

22.14 (B) Ranitidine does not affect the absorption of ciprofloxacin as do the other agents listed. (*10, pp 388–389*)

22.15 (B) Digoxin is mostly metabolized by the kidneys. Elderly patients or patients with renal disease and low creatinine clearance should be monitored carefully for signs of digoxin toxicity. (*11, p 989*)

22.16 (C) The H_2 receptor antagonists competitively inhibit the action of histamine on H_2 receptors in the stomach (e.g., acid production) without affecting the synthesis, release, or transformation of histamine. However, they are less effective than proton pump inhibitors (such as omeprazole) in reducing gastric acid secretion. (*1, p 308*)

22.17 (D) Loop diuretics favor excretion of potassium and hydrogen ions, thereby promoting hypokalemia and alkalosis. (*1, pp 218–219*)

22.18 (C) Enoxaparin, like heparin, requires the presence of the plasma serine protease inhibitor (antithrombin-III) and markedly increases its activity. It is used for the primary prevention of deep venous thrombosis (DVT) following hip replacement procedures. Warfarin (Coumadin) interferes with vitamin K synthesis. (*1, pp 207–210*)

22.19 (D) Erythromycin (the estolate form is better for children) is the first-line agent in the treatment of *B. pertussis;* trimethoprim/sulfamethoxazole is a second-line agent, and tetracycline and amoxicillin are third-line agents. (*1, p 248*)

22.20 (E) Although not well established, these effects of vitamin E have been reported. (*12, p 720*)

22.21 (D) Clonidine appears to work on α_2 receptors in the brainstem (probably the nucleus tractus solitarius) to decrease sympathetic outflow to the heart, kidneys, and blood vessels. (*1, p 184*)

22.22 (D) Ciprofloxacin targets the enzyme DNA gyrase, which is critical in DNA replication. Erythromycin acts at the level of ribosomes, while tircuoillin and vancomycin interfere with cell wall synthesis. (*1, pp 419–432*)

22.23 (A) Of the medications listed, only hydrochlorothiazide is not known to be ototoxic. (*1, p 412*)

22.24 (D) Each of the factors listed puts patients at risk of developing ototoxicity, especially when there is a history of pre-existing sensorineural hearing loss as with old age. (*1, p 413*)

22.25 (D) Clindamycin is a broad-spectrum agent that is considered very effective against mixed anaerobic-aerobic infections. (*1, p 435*)

22.26 (D) Tetracyclines are effective against a number of bacteria, including chlamydia, mycoplasma, spirochetes (e.g., Lyme disease), rickettsia, and *Legionella* species. They are not effective against *S. aureus,* particularly those strains that are methicillin resistant. (*1, p 436*)

22.27 (E) All three statements are correct. (*13, pp 34–35*)

22.28 (A) Rifampin stimulates hepatic metabolism of phenytoin, thereby decreasing its serum levels and favoring breakthrough seizures. However, INH interferes with Dilantin metabolism and tends to raise its serum levels; thus, the dose may not need to be adjusted. (*6, p 209*)

22.29 (C) Pyrimethamine (usually in combination with sulfadiazine) is used to treat toxoplasmosis. (*1, p 476*)

22.30 (B) INH is not active against so-called atypical mycobacteria such as *M. kansasii, Mycobacterium avium intracellulare* (MAI), and others. (*7, p 137*)

22.31 (B) Rifampin is used in combination with a β-lactam or with vancomycin to treat serious staph infections, particularly endocarditis and osteomyelitis. (*1, p 438*)

22.32 (A) Hypercalcemia is not an adverse effect of potassium-sparing diuretics such as spironolactone. (*6, p 412*)

22.33 (C) Kinins are hypotensive agents because of their vaso-dilatory effects on resistance vessels (e.g., arterioles). However, they constrict larger vessels, both arteries and veins, including umbilical vessels and the ductus arteriosus. (*15*, *p 294*)

22.34 (C) Vinblastine is an antimitotic agent, whereas methotrexate is an antimetabolite and bleomycin is an antibiotic. Cyclophosphamide is a nitrogen mustard type of agent that cross-links DNA. (*1, pp 508–522*)

22.35 (C) As with the case of α_2 adrenergic receptors, which regulate the release of norepinephrine, H_3 serves as an autoregulatory in the control of histamine release. (*15*, *p 262*)

22.36 (D) Losartan and other such drugs block the receptors for and thereby antagonize the effects of angiotensin II. These drugs are useful in treating hypertension and appear to work better in nonblack than black patients. (*16, p 4*)

22.37 (D) The bacteria most frequently encountered in the community (*Streptococcus pneumoniae, Haemophilus influenzae, Mycoplasma pneumoniae*, legionella, and chlamydia) can all be treated using a macrolide (erythromycin) or quinolone (levofloxacin) when the patient is less than 60 years old and has no comorbid conditions; amoxicillin/clavulanate (Augmentin) is more appropriate in older patients or patients with comorbid diseases. (*6, p 263*)

22.38 (E) Any of the factors listed is potentially a cause of adverse drug effects in the elderly. (*6, pp 402–403*)

22.39 (E) All three adverse reactions are associated with chronic NSAID use, especially in patients who are elderly. (*6, pp 431–432*)

22.40 (C) Estrogens are used to treat osteoporosis because of their anabolic effects on bone. (*9, p 177*)

22.41 (A) Adverse effects of isotretinoin (Acutane) are similar to those of hypervitaminosis A and include dryness of skin and mucous membranes and itching. Other adverse effects include alopecia, anorexia, headache, and others. The half-life of this agent is 10 to 20 h. (*17, p 1007*)

22.42 (A) Inflammation makes the tight junctions between astrocytes and pericytes and capillary endothelial cells more leaky, thus allowing ionized substances to gain access to the brain. (*18, p 819*)

22.43 (A) Azithromycin (Zithromax) has proven effective as a single agent and causes fewer cases of gastrointestinal problems. (*6, p 285*)

22.44 (D) Option A refers to phase I, B to phase II, and C to phase III. (*19, pp 62–72*)

22.45 (E) Each of the regimens listed is acceptable for the treatment of genital herpes as per 1998 CDC guidelines. (*20, pp 1–116*)

22.46 (D) Blood flow to an organ, the solubility of a drug, and whether or not it penetrates such barriers as the blood-brain barrier (BBB) all affect the effectiveness of a drug. (*1, p 70*)

22.47 (B) Phase II reactions are called synthetic, whereas phase I reactions are nonsynthetic. Methylation is carried out by a cytoplasmic transferase. (*1, pp 73–76*)

22.48 (C) A transdermal source of nicotine breaks the connection between the behavior of smoking and the effect of nicotine and provides for a smooth process of detoxification over a 2- to 3-wk period. (*1, p 548*)

22.49 (D) At the end of one half-life ($t_{1/2}$), i.e., 20 h, 50% of the drug is eliminated. At the end of the second half-life (i.e., 40 h), an additional 50% of the 50% left, or 25% of the original dose, is eliminated. Thus, by the end of 60 h (after three $t_{1/2}$s), 87.5% of the original dose is eliminated. (*1, pp 76–77*)

22.50 (E) Ergot alkaloids produce vasoconstriction, including vasoconstriction of veins, thus the contraindications. (*15, p 283*)

22.51 (D) Bromocriptine is extremely effective in lowering prolactin levels produced by anterior pituitary tumors, and is used to control physiologic lactation. (*15, p 282*)

22.52 (A) Tachyphylaxis refers to diminished responsiveness to a drug after its administration. Hypersensitivity usually refers to allergic or immunologic reactions to the drug. Hyperreactivity signifies that the intensity of the response to a drug is increased as compared to that seen in most patients. (*21, p 30*)

22.53 (D) Prazosin and its congeners reduce serum LDL in addition to reducing blood pressure and ameliorating CHF through peripheral-resistance-lowering action. (*1, p 185*)

22.54 (A) The difference between therapeutic and toxic levels in the case of digoxin is relatively small; thus the therapeutic index is narrow. This necessitates close monitoring of patients medicated with this drug. (*13, p 36*)

22.55 (B) The vasodilatory effect of nitroprusside is immediate. (*1, p 189*)

22.56 (E) Glucose intolerance is probably the best-known adverse effect of chronic corticosteroid use. Myopathy is due to the catabolic effects of these agents, and cataracts may represent both direct and indirect effects. (*6, p 225*)

22.57 (D) Reflex bradycardia is mediated by the vagus (cranial nerve X), which is interrupted during transplant. Therefore NE will not produce a reflex decrease in heart rate. (*22, p 84*)

22.58 (D) Tyramine causes the release of norepinephrine from the vesicles. (*22, p 86*)

22.59 (C) Erythromycin and related macrolides are used as alternate drugs for the penicillin-allergic patient. (*1, p 390*)

22.60 (D) The following are discontinued preoperatively. oral hypoglycemics, in order to avoid hypoglycemia; diuretics, to avoid hypovolemia and hypokalemia; and warfarin, to avoid excessive intraoperative bleeding. Antibiotics should be started to prevent wound infection. (*1, p 403*)

22.61 (E) At appropriately low doses, dopamine drip improves peripheral tissue perfusion, improves arterial pressure, and ameliorates oliguria. At high doses, dopamine exerts vasoconstrictive effects. (*23, pp 124–125*)

22.62 (E) Viagra is a vasodilator that ameliorates erectile dysfunction in patients with various problems. It has also been blamed for the deaths of many patients with cardiovascular disease requiring the use of nitrates because of synergistic effects. (*6, pp 121–123*)

22.63 (D) Atenolol and metoprolol are β-1 selective. Pindolol is nonselective. (*1, p 166*)

22.64 (B) Nitrates are used to decrease myocardial oxygen consumption principally by reducing preload. (*1, p 169*)

22.65 (C) Hypomagnesemia is the most likely explanation for cardiac sudden deaths following high doses of thiazides. (*6, p 369*)

22.66 (E) Diabetics, pregnant females, and patients with more than 7 days of symptoms of uncomplicated cystitis should receive a 7-day course of antimicrobials (such as Bactrim, if sulfa tolerant). Otherwise, a 3-day course is indicated. (*6, p 281*)

22.67 (D) Black patients do not respond well to beta blockers or ACE inhibitors. (*1, p 180*)

22.68 (D) Furosemide (Lasix) prevents calcium reabsorption by the renal tubules. Additionally, along with sodium, potassium, and magnesium loss through its diuretic activity, it promotes calciuria. (*1, p 219*)

22.69 (D) Calcium channel blockers are indicated for the treatment of essential hypertension, angina, and arrhythmias.

Both diltiazem and verapamil affect AV nodal conduction and may be used to slow conduction through the AV node. (*24, p 191*)

22.70 (A) Many different types of medications can be used, either alone or in combination, for the treatment of hypertension. Although a good antihypertensive medication, verapamil would not be a good choice in this situation because of its constipating effect. Amitriptyline (Elavil) also has anticholinergic effects that result in constipation. (*1, p 186*)

22.71 (D) Methadone is classified as an analgesic; the other three are stimulants. (*1, p 545*)

22.72 (E) SSRIs are better accepted by patients because of all the properties listed. (*1, p 111*)

22.73 (D) Nelfinavir (Viracept) is a protease inhibitor; the others are reverse transcriptase inhibitors. (*1, pp 456–458*)

22.74 (A) Amitriptyline has been found to ameliorate other pain conditions, but its main therapeutic action is to inhibit norepinephrine uptake. Propranolol, a nonselective beta blocker, is the most widely used migraine prophylactic medication; verapamil and ergotamine have also been found useful. (*15, p 282*)

22.75 (C) All four antifungals share the same action on fungal cells; they bind to sterols in the cell membrane, making it permeable to small molecules and rendering the cell susceptible to disruption. Only amphotericin B affects both host and fungal cells. (*1, pp 480–481*)

22.76 (D) The adverse effects of didanosine include peripheral neuropathy and pancreatitis. (*1, p 458*)

22.77 (D) Ganciclovir is similar to acyclovir both in term of structure and mechanism of action. Ganciclovir is indicated for CMV retinitis and other infections in immunocompromised patients. Foscarnet is active with a number of viruses including CMV, and is used when ganciclovir is not tolerated or not effective. Acyclovir is much less potent than ganciclovir. (*7, p 179*)

22.78 (C)   Saquinavir and similar drugs are protease inhibitors (PIs), which prevent the "packaging" of the viral components necessary prior to discharge of new viruses from infected CD4 cells. These agents are used in combination with other antiretrovirals. (*1, p 458*)

22.79 (A)   The interaction between glipizide and alcohol produces a disulfiram-like reaction. Patients taking glipizide are likely to develop hyperglycemia when thiazides are added to the regimen; those medicated with warfarin or cimetidine are more likely to develop hypoglycemia. (*9, p 135*)

22.80 (D)   Chronic alcoholism is a major cause of chronic pancreatitis in the United States. This patient is presenting with signs and symptoms of steatorrhea, which is due to maldigested food attributable to pancreatic lipase deficiency. (*1, p 316*)

References

1. Page CP, Curtis MJ, Sutter MC, et al: *Integrated Pharmacology,* St. Louis, Mosby, 1997.

2. Beck LH: A woman with drug resistant tuberculosis—Case study. *Phys Assist* 19(6):65, 1995.

3. Molavi A: Antimicrobials III: Macrolides, clindamycin, metronidazole, sulfonamides, trimethoprim, chloramphenicol, and tetracyclines. In: DiPalma JR, DiGregorio GJ, Barbieri EJ, Ferko AP (eds): *Basic Pharmacology in Medicine,* 4/e, West Chester, PA, Medical Surveillance, 1994.

4. Hoskins B: Antidepressant drugs. In: DiPalma JR, DiGregorio GJ, Barbieri EJ, Ferko AP (eds): *Basic Pharmacology in Medicine,* 4/e, West Chester, PA, Medical Surveillance, 1994.

5. Molavi A: Antimicrobials I: General concepts, beta-lactam antibiotics, and glycopeptides. In: DiPalma JR, DiGregorio GJ, Barbieri EJ, Ferko AP (eds): *Basic Pharmacology in Medicine,* 4/e, West Chester, PA, Medical Surveillance, 1994.

6. Bosker G: *Pharmatecture: Minimizing Medications to Maximize Results,* 2/e (revised), St. Louis, Facts and Comparisons, 1999.

7. *Physician Assistants' Prescribing Reference, Summer 2000.* New York, Prescribing Reference, 2000.

8. Benowitz NL: Antihypertensive agents. In: Katzung BG (ed): *Basic & Clinical Pharmacology,* 7/e, Stamford, CT, Appleton & Lange, 1998.

9. Grajeda-Higley L: *Understanding Pharmacology: A Physiologic Approach,* Stamford, CT, Appleton & Lange, 2000.

10. Lesse AJ: Miscellaneous agents: Quinolones, sulfonamides, and trimethoprim, urinary tract agents, metronidazole, spectinomycin, bacitracin, and antimycobacterial drugs. In: Smith CM, Reynard AM (eds): *Essentials of Pharmacology*, Philadelphia, Saunders, 1995.

11. Katzung BG: Special aspects of geriatric pharmacology. In: Katzung BG (ed): *Basic & Clinical Pharmacology*, 7/e, Stamford, CT, Appleton & Lange, 1998.

12. Schneider DR: Vitamins. In: DiPalma JR, DiGregorio GJ, Barbieri EJ, Ferko AP (eds): *Basic Pharmacology in Medicine*, 4/e, West Chester, PA, Medical Surveillance, 1994.

13. Holford NHG, Benet LZ: Pharmacokinetics and pharmacodynamics: Drug selection and the time course of drug action. In: Katzung BG (ed): *Basic & Clinical Pharmacology*, 7/e, Stamford, CT, Appleton & Lange, 1998.

14. Reid IA: Vasoactive peptides. In: Katzung BG (ed): *Basic & Clinical Pharmacology*, 7/e, Stamford, CT, Appleton & Lange, 1998.

15. Burkhalter A, Julius DA, Katzung BG: Histamine, serotonin, and the ergot alkaloids. In: Katzung BG (ed): *Basic & Clinical Pharmacology*, 7/e, Stamford, CT, Appleton & Lange, 1998.

16. *Physician Assistants' Prescribing Reference, Winter 1999–2000*, New York, Prescribing Reference, 1999.

17. Robertson DB, Maibach HI: Dermatologic pharmacology. In: Katzung BG (ed): *Basic & Clinical Pharmacology*, 7/e, Stamford, CT, Appleton & Lange, 1998.

18. Lampiris HW, Maddix DS: Clinical uses of antimicrobial agents. In: Katzung BG (ed): *Basic & Clinical Pharmacology*, 7/e, Stamford, CT, Appleton & Lange, 1998.

19. Berkowitz BA, Katzung BG: Basic and clinical evaluation of new drugs. In: Katzung BG (ed): *Basic & Clinical Pharmacology*, 7/e, Stamford, CT, Appleton & Lange, 1998.

20. Centers for Disease Control and Prevention: Guidelines for treatment of sexually transmitted diseases. *MMWR Morb Mort Wkly Rep* 47(RR-1):1–116, 1998.

21. Bourne, HR: Drug receptors and pharmacodynamics. In: Katzung BG (ed): *Basic & Clinical Pharmacology,* 7/e, Stamford, CT, Appleton & Lange, 1998.

22. Katzung BG: Introduction to autonomic pharmacology. In: Katzung BG (ed): *Basic & Clinical Pharmacology,* 7/e, Stamford, CT, Appleton & Lange, 1998.

23. Hoffman BB: Adrenoceptor-activating and other sympathomimetic drugs. In: Katzung BG (ed): *Basic & Clinical Pharmacology,* 7/e, Stamford, CT, Appleton & Lange, 1998.

24. Katzung BG, Chatterjee K: Vasodilators and the treatment of angina pectoris. In: Katzung BG (ed): *Basic & Clinical Pharmacology,* 7/e, Stamford, CT, Appleton & Lange, 1998.

23

Endocrinology

Salah Ayachi, PhD, PA-C

DIRECTIONS (Questions 23.1–23.21): Each of the numbered items or incomplete statements in this chapter is followed by answers or completions of the statement. Select the **one** lettered answer or completion that is **best** in each case.

23.1 Endometriosis (the presence of endometrial glands and stroma outside the uterine cavity) is common in women of childbearing age. Medical management of this condition is predicated on the knowledge that
  A. Estrogens stimulate growth of endometriosis.
  B. Progestins have an analgesic effect.
  C. Danazol reduces the midcycle surge of luteinizing hormone.
  D. A and B
  E. A, B, and C

23.2 Cutaneous manifestations of Graves' disease include the following
  A. Hyperhidrosis
  B. Pretibial edema
  C. Palmar erythema
  D. A and B
  E. A, B, and C

361

23.3 Which of the following is **NOT** true of pubertal growth?
  A. It is highly variable.
  B. It is partly influenced by adrenal hormones.
  C. It is partly influenced by gonadal hormones.
  D. It lasts 3 to 4 years.

23.4 In the workup of children of short stature, thyroid function must be evaluated. How is thyroid function best evaluated?
  A. Physical examination
  B. Thyroid scan
  C. Serum TSH level
  D. T_3 resin uptake

23.5 Estrogen replacement therapy (ERT) after menopause clearly has beneficial effects on many organ systems. Which of the following is adversely affected by ERT?
  A. Bone and fracture risk
  B. High-density lipoprotein levels
  C. Incidence of stroke
  D. Endometrial cancer risk

23.6 Whereas aging and dietary restriction have similar effects on the release of a number of hormones, they differ in others. Which hormone is decreased with aging and increased by dietary restriction?
  A. Thyroxine
  B. Insulin
  C. Luteinizing hormone
  D. Testosterone (in males)

23.7 Estrogens used for replacement therapy vary in potency, formulation, and source of origin. One preparation—conjugated equine estrogen, extracted from the urine of pregnant mares—stimulates binding proteins to a greater degree than native estrogens. This would be expected to make
  A. More biologically active estrogen available
  B. Therapy more likely to be successful
  C. Therapy more likely to be ineffective
  D. No difference in terms of biologic activity

23.8 Arginine vasopressin (AVP), in conjunction with angiotensin II, serves to regulate blood volume and osmolality. Arginine vasopressin
   A. Is similar to growth hormone
   B. Is bound to neurophysin II in the neurohypophysis
   C. Is released in higher quantities during the daytime
   D. Helps raise the renal medullary gradient

23.9 Diabetes insipidus (DI) is characterized by excretion of abnormally large volumes of urine and polydipsia. Several etiologies can account for this condition. Which of the known types is due to increased metabolism of AVP?
   A. Gestational DI
   B. Nephrogenic DI
   C. Cranial DI
   D. Dipsogenic DI

23.10 Many factors play important roles in growth. One of the more common causes of failure to grow in children is hypothyroidism. Which of the following reduces growth hormone secretion?
   A. Stress
   B. Exercise
   C. Hypoglycemia
   D. Psychological deprivation

23.11 Pregnancy-induced diabetes is due to a combination of insulin resistance and impaired secretion. A placental hormone that contributes to this is
   A. Progesterone
   B. Prolactin
   C. Cortisol
   D. Epinephrine

23.12 The majority of cases of primary hypothyroidism are
   A. Due to autoimmune (Hashimoto's) thyroiditis
   B. Postablative
   C. Drug induced
   D. Congenital

23.13 Our knowledge of cell membrane receptors and signaling processes has expanded over the last several years. This has added to our understanding of many disease states. Which of the following disease states is due to gain in function of receptors?
  A. Congenital hyperthyroidism
  B. Hirschsprung's disease
  C. Color blindness
  D. Nephrogenic diabetes insipidus

23.14 The brain is known to produce its own steroids, such as pregnenolone sulfate and dehydroepiandrosterone (DHEA). A steroid generated by brain tissue and described as important in the growth of Schwann cells and formation of myelin is
  A. Testosterone
  B. Estradiol
  C. Progesterone
  D. Cholesterol

23.15 A 42-year-old African American female complains of increasing fatigue over the past several months. Further history reveals weight gain, hoarseness of voice, and constipation. The patient has edema of both hands and face and xerosis (dry skin). This is a classic picture of
  A. Cushing's disease
  B. Acromegaly
  C. Hypothyroidism
  D. Graves' disease
  E. Addison's disease

23.16 Erythropoietin (Epo) is a glycoprotein hormone produced by renal tubular cells in response to hypoxia. In which of the following conditions has Epo been used most extensively?
  A. Anemia due to end-stage renal disease
  B. Anemia of zidovudine (AZT) therapy
  C. Anemia of prematurity
  D. Anemia of malignancy

23.17 Anemic patients, irrespective of etiology, have been found to respond to administration of

A. Glucocorticoids
B. Androgens
C. Thyroid hormone
D. A and B
E. A, B, and C

23.18 Interleukin-1, a peptide growth factor produced primarily by activated macrophages and other cells, has several known actions including all of the following **EXCEPT**
A. Pyrogenesis through action on the hypothalamus
B. Thyroid stimulation through TSH release
C. Glucocorticoid release through ACTH
D. Cardiac muscle hypertrophy

23.19 Patients with hypocalcemia due to chronic renal insufficiency may be treated with calcium supplements and given vitamin D_3 in some form. This is designed to
A. Reverse vitamin D_3 hypervitaminosis
B. Decrease serum calcium levels
C. Correct the hypocalcemic state induced by acidosis
D. A and B

23.20 Plasma ACTH levels are used to differentiate pituitary from adrenal causes of adrenal dysfunction. Which of the following is **INCORRECT?**
A. In primary adrenal insufficiency, ACTH levels are elevated.
B. In secondary adrenal insufficiency, ACTH levels may be so low as to be undetectable.
C. Plasma ACTH is markedly depressed in cases of congenital adrenal hyperplasia.
D. A and B
E. A and C

23.21 Adrenal insufficiency can be due to many different causes including fungal infections. Which fungal infection accounts for most cases of adrenal insufficiency in the U.S.?
A. Histoplasmosis
B. Coccidioidomycosis
C. Blastomycosis
D. Sporotrichosis

Endocrinology

Answers and Discussion

23.1 (E) Growth of endometriotic tissues is stimulated by estrogens and inhibited by danazol. Progestins, through their analgesic effect, are used to reduce the pain of endometriosis. (*1, pp 126–138*)

23.2 (E) Patients with Graves' disease present with all the manifestations listed. (*2, pp 12–17*)

23.3 (D) The pubertal growth spurt lasts only about 2 years and is accompanied by sexual development. (*3, pp 37–54*)

23.4 (C) Serum thyroid-stimulating hormone (TSH) level is the most convenient test of thyroid function. (*3, pp 37–54*)

23.5 (D) ERT helps maintain bone density, decreases the risk of future fractures, increases HDL cholesterol, and reduces the risk of stroke. However, it also increases the risk of endometrial cancer by up to 15-fold according to some reports. (*4, pp 492–509*)

23.6 (D) Aging and dietary restriction have been reported to decrease the production of thyroxine, insulin, and luteinizing hormone; dietary restriction increases testosterone production in males and aging decreases it. (*5, pp 61–93*)

23.7 (C) With stimulation of binding protein synthesis by non-native estrogens (e.g., equine estrogens), more estrogens will be bound by plasma proteins and make less biologically active (free) hormone available, thereby making therapy less likely to be successful. (*6, pp 161–179*)

23.8 (B) Arginine vasopressin (also known as antidiuretic hormone [ADH]) has a significant role in regulating serum osmolarity, volume, and fluid homeostasis. It is similar to oxytocin, is released in higher quantities at night (in older children), and is involved in concentrating the urine. In the neurohypophysis, it is bound to neurophysin II, which is thought to provide protection from degradation. (*7, pp 3–20*)

23.9 (A) Only gestational DI is attributable to increased metabolism of AVP. Nephrogenic, cranial, and dipsogenic DI are due to renal insensitivity to the hormone, destruction of the neurohypophysis, and excessive water intake, respectively. (*8, pp 21–38*)

23.10 (D) GH secretion is pulsatile and occurs during sleep or in the early A.M. hours. Psychological deprivation is known to inhibit GH secretion, whereas obesity reduces both the intensity and frequency of the peaks. The other factors listed increase GH secretion. (*9, pp 39–60*)

23.11 (A) Progesterone is secreted by the placenta. All others are produced elsewhere. (*10, pp 169–189*)

23.12 (A) Postablative (postsurgical or posttherapy for hyperthyroidism) hypothyroidism is the second most common type of hypothyroidism. Lithium and iodine-containing drugs account for a lesser proportion of hypothyroid cases. Congenital cases are rare. (*11, pp 107–118*)

23.13 (A) Congenital hyperthyroidism (autosomal dominant inheritance) is attributed to gain of TSH receptors resulting from mutation of G-protein-coupled receptors. The other conditions mentioned are reportedly due to loss of function of their respective receptors. (*12, pp 9–33*)

23.14 (C) Progesterone plays an important role in the growth of Schwann cells and the formation of myelin. It is among several steroids that neural tissue produces locally. (*13, pp 63–78*)

23.15 (C) Hypothyroidism affects all body systems. With decreased levels of thyroid hormones, energy metabolism and heat production are decreased; the individual complains of cold intolerance, lethargy, tiredness, and weight gain. Further, there is an increased amount of protein and mucopolysaccharides that bind water, producing nonpitting edema as well as thickening of the tongue and of laryngopharyngeal mucous membranes and contributing to hoarseness and slurring of speech. (*14, pp 1104–1106*)

23.16 (A) Relative deficiency of Epo is the main problem in end-stage renal disease, and Epo administration has been found effective in ameliorating anemia-related symptoms in patients with this condition. (*15, p 1238*)

23.17 (E) The hormones listed all have beneficial effects in anemic patients and appear to act mostly through Epo. (*16, pp 58–59*)

23.18 (D) Although interleukin-1 has been reported to stimulate smooth muscle activity, there is no indication that it has any direct stimulatory action on cardiomyocytes. (*17, pp 115–128*)

23.19 (C) Chronic renal insufficiency leads to acidosis, which favors calciuria and hypocalcemia (the kidneys are no longer able to reabsorb adequate calcium to maintain normal serum levels). Supplemental calcium and vitamin D_3 are given to reverse these changes. (*18, p 900*)

23.20 (C) In primary adrenal insufficiency, the diseased adrenal is unresponsive to ACTH; in secondary adrenal dysfunction, the pituitary production of ACTH is inadequate. In the six common forms of congenital adrenal hyperplasia, adrenal production of cortisol is defective, leading to increased ACTH production and adrenal hyperplasia. (*19, pp 317–358*)

23.21 **(B)** The most common cause of fungal-induced adrenal insufficiency in the U.S. is *Histoplasma capsulatum.* Worldwide, the major cause is tuberculosis. (*20, pp 1463–1475*)

References

1. Tarnay CM, DeCherney AH: Update on endometriosis: Medical therapy, surgery, or both? *Women's Health Prim Care* 2(2):126–138, 1999.

2. McTigue J: Cutaneous manifestations of thyroid disorders. *JAAPA* 11(4):12–17, 1998.

3. Wesoly S, Saenger P: Evaluation and treatment of short stature in children. *JAAPA* 11(4):37–54, 1998.

4. Villareal DT, Morley JE: Trophic factors in aging. Should older people receive hormonal replacement therapy? *Drugs Aging* 4:492–509, 1994.

5. Morley JE: Aging. In: Bagdale JW (ed): *Yearbook of Endocrinology,* St. Louis, Mosby, 1993.

6. Notelovitz M: Menopause. In: Morley JE, van den Berg L (eds): *Contemporary Endocrinology: Endocrinology of Aging,* Totowa, NJ, Humana, 2000.

7. Zimmerman D, Uramoto G: Diabetes insipidus in pediatrics. In: Meikle AW (ed): *Contemporary Endocrinology: Hormone Replacement Therapy,* Totowa, NJ, Humana, 1999.

8. Drincic AT, Robertson GL: Treatment of diabetes insipidus in adults. In: Meikle AW (ed): *Contemporary Endocrinology: Hormone Replacement Therapy,* Totowa, NJ, Humana, 1999.

9. Lum CK, Wilson DM: Growth hormone therapy in children. In: Meikle AW (ed). *Contemporary Endocrinology: Hormone Replacement Therapy,* Totowa, NJ, Humana, 1999.

10. McFarland KF, Irwin LS: Management of diabetes in pregnancy. In: Meikle AW (ed): *Contemporary Endocrinology:*

Hormone Replacement Therapy, Totowa, NJ, Humana, 1999.

11. Cooper DS: Thyroid hormone replacement therapy for primary and secondary hypothyroidism. In: Meikle AW (ed): *Contemporary Endocrinology: Hormone Replacement Therapy,* Totowa, NJ, Humana, 1999.

12. Mayo KE: Receptors: Molecular mediators of hormone action. In: Conn PM, Melmed S (eds): *Endocrinology: Basic and Clinical Principles,* Totowa, NJ, Humana, 1997.

13. McEwen BS: Hormone actions in the brain. In: Conn PM, Melmed S (eds): *Endocrinology: Basic and Clinical Principles,* Totowa, NJ, Humana, 1997.

14. Fitzgerald PA: Endocrinology. In: Tierney LM Jr, McPhee SJ, Papadakis MA (eds): *Current Medical Diagnosis & Treatment,* 39/e, New York, McGraw-Hill, 2000.

15. Huether SE: Alterations of hormonal regulation. In McCance KL, Huether SE (eds): *Pathophysiology: The Biologic Basis for Disease in Adults and Children,* 3/e, St. Louis, Mosby, 1998.

16. Grossi A, Vannucchi AM, Rafanelli D, Ferrini PR: The humoral regulation of normal and pathologic erythropoiesis. In: Foa PP (ed): *Humoral Factors in the Regulation of Tissue Growth: Blood, Blood Vessels, Skeletal System and Teeth,* New York, Springer-Verlag, 1993.

17. Spangelo BL: Cytokines and endocrine function. In: Conn PM, Melmed S (eds): *Endocrinology: Basic and Clinical Principles,* Totowa, NJ, Humana, 1997.

18. Watnick S, Morrison G: Kidney. In: Tierney LM Jr, McPhee SJ, Papadakis, MA (eds): *Current Medical Diagnosis & Treatment,* 39/e, New York, McGraw-Hill, 2000.

19. Findling JW, Aron DC, Tyrrell JB: Glucocorticoids and adrenal androgens. In Greenspan FS, Baxter JD (eds): *Basic*

& *Clinical Endocrinology,* 4/e, Stamford, CT, Appleton & Lange, 1998.

20. Hamill RJ: Infectious diseases: Mycotic. In: Tierney LM Jr, McPhee SJ, Papadakis, MA (eds): *Current Medical Diagnosis & Treatment,* 39/e, New York, McGraw-Hill, 2000.

24

Fluid and Electrolyte Disorders

Salah Ayachi, PhD, PA-C, and Timothy F. Quigley, MS, PA-C

DIRECTIONS (Questions 24.1–24.28): Each of the numbered items or incomplete statements in this chapter is followed by answers or completions of the statement. Select the **one** lettered answer or completion that is **best** in each case.

24.1 Which of the following is true of the mechanism of action of mannitol in producing osmotic diuresis?
  A. It is metabolized by renal tubular cells, thereby producing acidosis.
  B. It acts as a loop diuretic.
  C. It is filtered, but not reabsorbed.
  D. It is effective when given orally.

24.2 Drugs that require dosage adjustment in patients with renal failure include
  A. Penicillins
  B. Digitalis
  C. Amphotericin B
  D. All of the above

24.3 The many causes of renal failure are classified as prerenal, intrarenal, and postrenal. Which of the following is considered intrarenal?
   A. Post-streptococcal glomerulonephritis
   B. Congestive heart failure (CHF)
   C. Benign prostatic hypertrophy (BPH)
   D. Renal vein thrombosis

24.4 Atrial natriuretic factor (also called atrial natriuretic peptide [ANP]), secreted by the atria in response to stress, decreases
   A. Glomerular filtration rate
   B. Release of aldosterone
   C. Release of antidiuretic hormone (ADH)
   D. Vasomotor tone

24.5 Signs and symptoms of fluid volume deficit (FVD) or hypovolemia include all of the following **EXCEPT**
   A. Orthostatic hypotension
   B. Poor skin turgor
   C. Decreased temperature
   D. Thirst

24.6 Isotonic saline solution (0.9% NaCl) may be used to expand intravascular volume and replace extracellular fluid (ECF). One drawback to the use of isotonic saline is that it
   A. Cannot be administered with blood products
   B. Does not provide free water, calories, or other electrolytes
   C. Must be administered slowly
   D. May cause hyperchloremic acidosis

24.7 Risk factors for development of hypervolemia include
   A. Heart failure
   B. Cirrhosis
   C. Nephrotic syndrome
   D. A and B
   E. A, B, and C

24.8 Edema may develop when there is alteration in capillary hemodynamics resulting in either increased formation or decreased removal of interstitial fluid (ISF). Which of the

following favors increased capillary permeability and formation of ISF?
A. Allergy
B. Lymphatic obstruction
C. Liver failure
D. Heart failure

24.9 Complications of diuretic therapy include all of the following **EXCEPT**
A. Volume depletion
B. Hyperkalemia
C. Hypokalemia
D. Hypermagnesemia

24.10 Which of the following is **NOT** an etiology of isotonic fluid volume deficit (FVD)?
A. Hemorrhage
B. Lack of intake of fluid and electrolytes
C. Vomiting
D. Osmotic diuresis

24.11 Sodium deficiency (hyponatremia) usually develops with all of the following **EXCEPT**
A. Prolonged diuretic therapy
B. Excessive diaphoresis
C. Prolonged vomiting
D. Diabetes insipidus

24.12 Which of the following solutions should be administered intravenously to a hyponatremic patient?
A. Lactated Ringer's
B. Isotonic (0.9% NaCl) saline
C. Hypertonic (3% NaCl) saline
D. Hypotonic (0.45% NaCl) saline

24.13 Patients with inadequate renal function and severe hyperglycemia present with expanded ECF because of
   A. Water shift from ICF to ECF
   B. Electrolytes and water not being lost during osmotic diuresis
   C. Oliguria with end-stage renal disease (ESRD)
   D. All of the above

24.14 A patient in uncompensated respiratory acidosis would have all of the following **EXCEPT**
   A. $pH < 7.35$
   B. $Paco_2 > 40$ mm Hg
   C. $HCO_3 = 18$ m Eq/L
   D. A and B

24.15 In assessing a patient for metabolic acidosis, you would expect him or her to have
   A. Hypokalemia
   B. Tetany
   C. Kussmaul breathing
   D. $pH > 4.5$

24.16 Hyponatremia (serum Na less than 130 mEq/L) may be caused by many different disease states. Which of the following is **NOT** associated with hyponatremia?
   A. Congestive heart failure
   B. Hyperparathyroidism
   C. Lymphoma
   D. Pancreatitis

24.17 Complications of diuretic use include all the following **EXCEPT**
   A. Hypermagnesemia
   B. Hypokalemia
   C. Hyponatremia
   D. Metabolic alkalosis

24.18 Causes of euvolemic hypotonic hyponatremia include all of the following **EXCEPT**
   A. Dehydration
   B. Postoperative complications

C. Psychogenic polydipsia
D. Syndrome of inappropriate ADH secretion

24.19 Causes of hypernatremia include all of the following **EXCEPT**
A. Excessive sweating without water replacement
B. Exertional losses from respiratory tract
C. Idiosyncratic ACE inhibitor reaction
D. Nephrogenic diabetes insipidus

24.20 Recognized complications of diuretic use include all the following **EXCEPT**
A. Hyperkalemia
B. Hyponatremia
C. Metabolic alkalosis
D. Volume depletion

24.21 A grave danger of too rapid overcorrection of hyponatremia is irreversible central pontine myelinosis. To prevent this complication, the goal of therapy is to raise the serum sodium at a rate of
A. 0.5 mEq/L/h
B. 1.0 mEq/L/h
C. 2.0 mEq/L/h
D. 3.0 mEq/L/h

24.22 Signs and symptoms of hypokalemia include all of the following **EXCEPT**
A. Constipation
B. Fatigue
C. Hyperreflexia
D. Muscle cramps

24.23 Which of the following is **NOT** an ECG manifestation of hypokalemia?
A. Decreased T wave amplitude
B. Elevated ST segment
C. Premature ventricular contraction
D. U wave

24.24 Which of the following statements about disorders of potassium metabolism is **FALSE?**
  A. The most common cause of hypokalemia is use of diuretics or laxatives.
  B. Aggressive IV potassium replacement is the treatment of choice in hypokalemia.
  C. Diabetic ketoacidosis is the most common cause of hyperkalemia.
  D. ACE inhibitor drugs can lead to the development of hyperkalemia.

24.25 All of the following represent possible etiologies of hypercalcemia **EXCEPT**
  A. Hypomagnesemia
  B. Immobilization
  C. Metastatic bone lesions
  D. Primary hyperparathyroidism

24.26 Which of the following **IS** a sign or symptom of hypocalcemia?
  A. Hypertension
  B. Neuropsychiatric symptoms
  C. Renal stones
  D. Seizures/tetany

24.27 All of the following are likely etiologies of hypomagnesemia **EXCEPT**
  A. Alcoholism with poor nutrition
  B. Aminoglycoside antibiotics
  C. Diuretics
  D. Renal insufficiency

24.28 Which of the following statements about phosphate metabolism is **FALSE?**
  A. Hyperphosphatemia is a rare disorder except in patients with chronic renal failure.
  B. Phosphate levels in growing children are typically higher than the normal adult range.
  C. Alcoholism and nutritional depletion are common causes of hypophosphatemia.
  D. Rapid correction of hypophosphatemia is the treatment of choice.

Fluid and Electrolyte Disorders

Answers and Discussion

24.1 (C) Mannitol is used to produce osmotic diuresis. It is not absorbed to any extent and is therefore ineffective if given orally. Furthermore, it is not a loop diuretic. It is effective when given intravenously since it is filtered and not reabsorbed. (*1, p 219*)

24.2 (D) Amphotericin B is an antifungal agent that is known to be nephrotoxic. Penicillins and digitalis drugs are excreted by the kidneys. Any patient with compromised renal function who must be given these medications will require careful monitoring and dose adjustment. (*2, p 223*)

24.3 (A) Renal failure resulting from strep infection is due to parenchymal damage to the glomerular structure. CHF and renal vein thrombosis are conditions that begin outside the kidneys per se. BPH may produce mechanical obstruction distal to the kidneys. (*2, pp 220–221*)

24.4 (A) ANP increases sodium and water excretion by increasing GFR as well as by decreasing aldosterone and ADH release and direct vasodilation. (*2, pp 19–20*)

24.5 (C) With FVD, blood pressure decreases especially upon standing. Skin turgor decreases, leading to tenting, and the patient complains of pain. However, body temperature rises. (*2, p 51*)

24.6 (D) Isotonic saline does not provide other electrolytes, calories, or free water, but it may be administered with blood products and infused without fear of significant alterations in intercompartment fluxes. However, it may cause hyperchloremic acidosis. (*2, pp 58–59*)

24.7 (E) In both heart failure and cirrhosis, there is a chronic stimulus to the kidneys to retain sodium and water. In nephrotic syndrome, renal function is decreased, leading to decreased sodium and water. (*2, pp 66–69*)

24.8 (A) Lymphatic channel obstruction increases ISF pressure and reduces drainage. Liver failure leads to decreased plasma oncotic pressure favoring extravasation into ISF spaces. In heart failure, venous and capillary pressures are increased. In allergy, histamine increases capillary permeability and promotes collection of fluids in the ISF spaces. (*2, pp 74–75*)

24.9 (D) Potassium-sparing diuretics predispose to hyperkalemia, while others, such as furosemide and thiazides, favor hypokalemia. Diuretics promote the loss of magnesium in the urine and hypomagnesemia. (*2, pp 76–80*)

24.10 (D) Osmotic diuresis is an etiology of hypertonic FVD. All others lead to isotonic FVD. (*3, pp 28–32*)

24.11 (D) Diabetes insipidus causes excessive loss of water with some electrolyte loss. Prolonged diuretic therapy causes impaired sodium reabsorption, and excessive sweating results in the loss of large amounts of sodium. (*3, pp 52–54*)

24.12 (C) Hypertonic saline should be infused carefully to replenish sodium in the ECF over an appropriate period of time so as to correct the disturbance slowly without precipitating neurologic changes. All others are not appropriate. (*4, p 233*)

24.13 (D) The extra load of glucose in the ECF causes osmotic diuresis and contraction of the ECF which, in turn, cause water to shift from ICF to ECF. With renal failure, especially if severe enough to be ESRD, there is little diuresis because of compromised GFR; therefore, water and electrolytes are not lost. (*5, pp 262–266*)

24.14 (C) In cases of uncompensated respiratory acidosis, the bicarbonate level is usually normal (24 mEq/L). (*3, p 115*)

24.15 (C) Hypokalemia, tetany, and a pH greater than 7.45 are associated with metabolic alkalosis. Kussmaul respirations are a finding in metabolic acidosis. (*3, pp 118–121*)

24.16 (B) Hyponatremia occurs in patients with increased extracellular fluid volume, such as in congestive heart failure, cirrhosis, or renal failure; in decreased extracellular fluid volume, such as gastrointestinal losses from vomiting, diarrhea, diuretics, pancreatitis, and burns; and in normal extracellular fluid volume, such as in hypothyroidism, SIADH of malignancy, and pulmonary and CNS disorders. Primary hyperparathyroidism is a common cause of hypercalcemia. (*6, p 1333*)

24.17 (A) Diuretic use can cause volume depletion, hypokalemia, hyponatremia, and metabolic alkalosis. Loop diuretics (furosemide, bumetanide, ethacrynic acid) produce the greatest diuresis in the shortest time and are active in the luminal side of the renal tubular epithelium. Thiazide diuretics (hydrochlorothiazide, chlorthalidone, metolazone) are less potent agents and are active in the proximal portions of the nephron. Hypermagnesemia is rarely seen in clinical practice except in patients receiving supplemental magnesium for toxemia of pregnancy or in patients with renal failure who use magnesium-containing antacids. (*6, pp 1334, 1337*)

24.18 (A) Dehydration is more often seen in the presence of hypernatremia. The diagnosis of hyponatremia of SIADH can only be made if the patient is euvolemic, because hypovolemia physiologically stimulates ADH secretion. Patients who develop hyponatremia in the postoperative period have often received excessive hypotonic fluid. Patients with bipolar disorder or other psychological problems may present with psychogenic polydipsia through excess free water intake and renal excretion of sodium to maintain euvolemia. (*7, pp 839–843*)

24.19 (C) Hypernatremia is rare in the presence of an intact thirst mechanism. Excess water loss (through diarrhea, exercise, dehydration, or nephrogenic diabetes insipidus) that is not replaced by appropriate water intake can lead to hypernatremia. The treatment of hypernatremia thus focuses on replacement of body water. However, too rapid correction can lead to cerebral edema and possible neurologic impairment. (*7, pp 843–844*)

24.20 (A) High-potency loop diuretics (such as furosemide) and lower-potency thiazide diuretics (such as hydrochlorothiazide) are commonly used in the presence of hypertension and edema. The most common complications of diuretic use are volume depletion, hypokalemia, hyponatremia, and metabolic alkalosis. (*6, p 1334*)

24.21 (B) Because of the potential for irreversible neurologic injury, hyponatremia therapy with hypertonic saline solutions should be reserved for those patients with neurologic symptoms. The treatment of choice in hyponatremia is to treat the underlying cause and to restrict water to less than 2 L daily. This conservative regimen is usually enough for patients without neurologic symptoms. If IV hypertonic saline is used, the goal should be to increase serum sodium up to 120 mEq/L at no more than 1 mEq/L/h. (*6, p 1333; 7, p 843*)

24.22 (C) Hyporeflexia, not hyperreflexia, is symptomatic of hypokalemia. In mild to moderate hypokalemia, the patient may present with muscle weakness, fatigue, and muscle cramps. In severe hypokalemia (<2.5 mEq/L), hyporeflexia, tetany, and flaccid paralysis may be present. Constipation or ileus may be seen in smooth muscle involvement. (*7, pp 844–845*)

24.23 (B) A depressed, not elevated, ST segment is typical of the ECG in hypokalemia. The likelihood of digitalis toxicity is also increased with hypokalemia. (*7, p 844*)

24.24 (B) Hypokalemia usually represents gastrointestinal or urinary potassium excretion. Since both laxative and diuretic use and abuse are so common in hypokalemia, health care providers need to consider surreptitious use in patients in whom another cause of hypokalemia is not apparent. Aggressive IV potassium replacement, however, can be dangerous in those with renal impairment or diabetes, and the concentrated IV solutions are caustic and painful when administered via peripheral veins. Ironically, ACE inhibitors are often recommended for slowing the progression of diabetic nephropathy, but since they can lead to hyperkalemia, both patients and providers need to be alert for such manifestations. Diabetic ketoacidosis, caused by the shifting of potassium from the intracellular to the extracellular space, is the most common cause of significant hyperkalemia. (*6, pp 1335–1336*)

24.25 (D) Asymptomatic hypercalcemia is most commonly attributable to primary hyperparathyroidism. If normal phosphate levels are found in the workup of hypercalcemia, metastatic bone lesions must be suspected. Vitamin D or vitamin A excess, multiple myeloma, thiazide diuretics, Paget's disease, and prolonged immobilization may also cause hypercalcemia. While hypophosphatemia may cause hypercalcemia, hypomagnesemia is a risk factor for hypocalcemia, not hypercalcemia. (*6, pp 1336–1337*)

24.26 (D) Signs and symptoms of hypocalcemia (seizures, muscle cramps, tetany, laryngospasm, abdominal pain, and paresthesias of the lips and extremities) are caused by excitation of neuromuscular and cardiovascular nerve and muscle cells. ECG changes are typified by prolongation of the QT interval. Signs and symptoms of hypercalcemia are most commonly polyuria and constipation, hypertension, stupor or coma, ventricular extrasystoles, and a shortened QT interval on ECG. Renal stones can also be caused by hypercalcemia. (*7, p 849*)

24.27 (D) Renal insufficiency in patients who use magnesium-containing antacids or laxatives is the primary cause of hypermagnesemia. Causes of hypomagnesemia include large volumes of IV fluids, diuretics, chemotherapeutic cisplatin, nephrotoxic antibiotics such as amphotericin B and aminoglycosides, and malnutrition with alcoholism. (*6, p 1337; 7, pp 852–853*)

24.28 (D) Hyperphosphatemia is a routine finding in the presence of chronic renal failure, but it is otherwise a rare finding. Since phosphate is an integral component of bone formation, levels of it are commonly higher in growing children than in adults. Malabsorption from small bowel bypass, malnutrition associated with alcoholism, diuretics use, and vitamin D deficiency may all cause hypophosphatemia. Rapid correction of hypophosphatemia is contraindicated because of the risk of hypocalcemia, and a frequently coexisting magnesium deficit should be treated simultaneously. (*6, p 1337; 7, pp 850–851*)

References

1. Star RA: Pathogenesis of diabetes insipidus and other polyuric states. In: Seldin DW, Giebisch G (eds): *Clinical Disturbances of Water Metabolism,* New York, Raven, 1993.

2. Horne MM, Swearingen PL: *Pocket Guide to Fluids, Electrolytes and Acid-Base Balance,* 2/e, St. Louis, Mosby-Year Book, 1993.

3. Paradiso C: Alterations in body fluid balance. In: *Lippincott's Review Series—Fluids and Electrolytes,* Philadelphia, Lippincott, 1995.

4. Sterns RH, Clark EC, Silver SM: Clinical consequences of hyponatremia and its correction. In: Seldin DW, Giebisch G (eds): *Clinical Disturbances of Water Metabolism,* New York, Raven, 1993.

5. Halperin ML, Goguen JM, Scheich AM, Kamel KS: Clinical consequences of hyperglycemia and its correction. In: Seldin DW, Giebisch G (eds): *Clinical Disturbances of Water Metabolism,* New York, Raven, 1993.

6. Bicknell SL, McCallum O, Wright LF: Urinary tract disorders. In: Rakel RE (ed): *Textbook of Family Practice,* 5/e, Philadelphia, Saunders, 1995.

7. Okuda T, Kurokawa K, Papadakis MA: Fluid and electrolyte disorders. In: Tierney LM, McPhee SJ, Papadakis MA (eds): *Current Medical Diagnosis & Treatment,* 38/e, Stamford, CT, Appleton & Lange, 1999.

25

Health Promotion and Disease Prevention

Barbara A. Lyons, MEd, PA-C

DIRECTIONS (Questions 25.1–25.20): Each of the numbered items or incomplete statements in this chapter is followed by answers or completion of the statement. Select the **one** lettered answer or completion that is **best** in each case.

25.1 A 48-year-old Taiwanese man comes to your office concerned about the possibility of having diabetes mellitus. He listened to a radio program about diabetes and became concerned about his own risk. His mother is 68 years old and has atherosclerosis and osteoarthritis; his father is 72 years old and has hypertension and diminished vision and hearing. Both of the patient's parents are from Taiwan. The patient's vital signs are as follows: pulse, 82 and regular; blood pressure, 128/86; respirations, 12 per minute and regular. His height is 5 ft, 8 in. (68 in.) and his weight is 141 lb. According to the U.S. Preventive Services Task Force, the patient meets which of the criteria placing him at high risk for diabetes mellitus?

A. Age

B. Ethnicity

C. Family history
D. Obesity
E. None of the criteria

25.2 A 52-year-old Caucasian woman comes to your clinic for an annual checkup. She moved from another state 2 years ago and is just getting around to making her initial contact with medical care in your town. She has never been pregnant and has no previous medical problems other than occasional upper respiratory infections. Which cancers would this patient be at risk for due to her history?
A. Ovarian
B. Breast
C. Both
D. Neither

25.3 A 22-year-old PA student is having the required yearly TB skin testing at the hospital where he is doing his clinical rotations. He does not have any known recent exposure to patients with TB and is otherwise healthy. A Mantoux test is placed on his forearm and read in 48 to 72 h. Erythema is measured at 15 mm. The appropriate clinical decision based on this information is to
A. Place another Mantoux test on the other forearm
B. Treat with isoniazid for prevention of TB infection
C. Place the patient on a multidrug antitubercular regimen
D. Remeasure the test results
E. Reassure the patient that he does not have TB

25.4 Varicella vaccine is generally given to children. Which of the following should receive the vaccine?
A. Nonpregnant women of childbearing age
B. Elementary school teachers
C. Both
D. Neither

25.5 Today, most authorities endorse using body mass index (BMI) to evaluate healthy weight for adults. The upper boundary for healthy weight is generally considered to be a BMI of
   A. 19
   B. 21
   C. 25
   D. 28
   E. Greater than 30

25.6 In your practice, you are assigned to evaluate potential student athletes for athletic participation. Which of the following patients may **NOT** be cleared for athletics?
   A. A 16-year-old boy with insulin-dependent diabetes mellitus who wants to play football
   B. A 13-year-old girl with moderate asthma who wants to play tennis
   C. A 15-year-old boy with a history of well-controlled seizure disorder who wants to wrestle
   D. A 12-year-old girl with HIV who wants to run track
   E. A 17-year-old boy who has carditis and wants to play soccer

25.7 Patients who smoke cigarettes often realize they are at higher risk for lung cancer. They may be surprised to know they are also at higher risk for
   A. Urinary bladder cancer
   B. Pancreatic cancer
   C. Both
   D. Neither

25.8 Which of the following does **NOT** affect the results of a guaiac stool test?
   A. Aspirin and/or nonsteroidal anti-inflammatory drugs
   B. Dietary iron supplements
   C. Iodine-containing anal preparations
   D. Vitamin E less than 250 mg per day

25.9 A 32-year-old Hispanic man comes to your office for a blood pressure check. Today is his third consecutive blood pressure reading. The average of the three readings is

152/96. The patient, who is about 20 lb overweight, does not exercise, drinks three or four beers per evening, and eats at fast food restaurants at which he consistently adds salt to his food. Your recommendations include all of the following **EXCEPT**

A. Beginning a low-intensity aerobic exercise program, i.e., walking
B. Losing weight
C. Reducing alcohol to no more than two drinks per day
D. Reducing sodium intake
E. Taking a diuretic for drug therapy

25.10 A 40-year-old woman desires to have her cholesterol level checked. Which of the following is a consideration that should be taken when performing her cholesterol screening?

A. She should be put on a special diet prior to testing, then fast completely for 12 h prior to the test.
B. Make sure to check her history for medication intake, since cholesterol levels may be decreased by intake of certain drugs such as bile salts, steroids, and progestins.
C. Screening is advisable if she is acutely ill, losing weight, pregnant, or nursing.
D. Testing is preferably done on a fingerstick sample of blood.
E. The sample should be taken only after the patient has been in the sitting position for at least 5 min.

25.11 Common wooden-shafted culture swabs are not used for chlamydia screening because

A. They usually have cotton tips, and cotton is not appropriate for the procurement of cells for testing.
B. The distance the swab tip must penetrate for cervical and urethral cultures is deeper, so the swab has to be of a smaller caliber.
C. These swabs do not have Dacron tips, which are considered the best for cell procurement.
D. Some woods contain substances that are toxic to chlamydia.

25.12 A 43-year-old man has been in a monogamous relationship for 10 years with his 39-year-old wife, who is 5 mo pregnant with their second child. A few days after engaging in unprotected vaginal intercourse with another woman, the man notices a discharge from his penis and is diagnosed by his PA as having gonorrhea. The patient is at risk for which other sexually transmitted disease(s)?
A. Chlamydia
B. Syphilis
C. Both
D. Neither

25.13 Upon further questioning, you find that the patient in question 25.12 has never had any form of hepatitis, nor has he been vaccinated for hepatitis B. The next step in the treatment plan for hepatitis B prophylaxis would be to
A. Administer hepatitis B immunoglobulin (HBIgG) only
B. Administer the hepatitis B vaccine series
C. Administer one dose of HBIgG and initiate the hepatitis B vaccine series
D. Depending on the other woman's hepatitis B status, contact and test her
E. Provide no treatment

25.14 When the corneal reflections of a light shone on the eyes do not fall symmetrically on corresponding points on the patient's corneas, the patient is said to have
A. Binocular depth perception abnormality
B. Decreased visual acuity
C. Strabismus
D. Astigmatism
E. Papilledema

25.15 There is evidence that the normal cutoff levels for hemoglobin and hematocrit in children older than 1 year are changed by all of the following factors **EXCEPT**
A. Age
B. Altitude
C. Ethnicity
D. Gender
E. Smoking

25.16 A 72-year-old white woman decides that she needs to find out if she has osteoporosis. Which of the following tests can discriminate between cortical and trabecular bone?
   A. Single photon absorption (SPA)
   B. Dual photon absorption (DPA)
   C. Dual energy x-ray absorption (DXA)
   D. Quantitative computed tomography (QCT)

25.17 A 24-year-old woman comes to your clinic for a preconception visit as she and her husband are thinking about starting a family within the next year. The woman is healthy with no allergies, but her blood work shows that she has an undetectable level of rubella antibodies. What should the course of action be?
   A. Immunize her with rubella only, measles-rubella, or measles-mumps-rubella vaccine.
   B. Advise her that there is no reason she cannot try to get pregnant right away.
   C. Give the vaccine intramuscularly.
   D. Advise her that the most common reaction to the immunization is low-grade fever.

25.18 Pneumococcal vaccine (Pneumovax) is **NOT** indicated in which of the following patients?
   A. A well 75-year-old woman who lives in her own home
   B. A frail 80-year-old man who lives in a nursing home and uses a walker for ambulation
   C. A 21-year-old gang member who had a knife wound to his belly and subsequent hepatorraphy and splenectomy
   D. A 25-year-old African American man who has had sickle cell disease all his life
   E. A 45-year-old woman who is hepatitis B antibody positive

25.19 A 70-year-old man is seeing a new health care provider as he has recently moved from his hometown in a large northern U.S. city to one of the southern states to take advantage of its warmer climate. You are to discuss the reasons why you have to do screening for prostate cancer during your screening physical. According to the U.S. Task Force, which of the following statements is **TRUE**?
  A. Screening for prostate cancer at this patient's age is not controversial.
  B. Assessment for prostatic acid phosphatase is the best test to use.
  C. Examining the patient's prostate via digital rectal examination is necessary.
  D. Watchful waiting and radical prostatectomy have not been shown to be any different in predicting mortality from prostate cancer.

25.20 At which age is it appropriate for children to begin drinking cow's milk?
  A. 6 mo
  B. 9 mo
  C. 12 mo
  D. 18 mo
  E. 24 mo

Health Promotion and Disease Prevention

Answers and Discussion

25.1 (E) The patient would have to be both over 40 and obese to meet the criteria for high risk of diabetes mellitus. (*1, p 273*)

25.2 (C) Nulliparity is a risk factor for both ovarian cancer and breast cancer. Being over 50 years old places this patient at risk for breast cancer due to age alone. (*1, p 207*)

25.3 (D) The Mantoux test is measured at the borders of induration, not erythema. The treatment classifications are based on this measurement. (*1, p 311*)

25.4 (C) Anyone who lives or works in a setting where varicella transmission is possible is a candidate for the varicella vaccine. This includes nonpregnant women (who should avoid getting pregnant for 1 mo after receiving the vaccine), teachers of young children, day care workers, college students, and people in the military. (*1, pp 116–120*)

25.5 (C) A BMI greater than 25 is considered pathognomonic for significant increase of mortality. (*1, p 196*)

25.6 (E) The presence of carditis may result in sudden death on exertion. Athletes with fever should also be precluded from participation, as it can increase cardiopulmonary effort, reduce maximum exercise capacity, make heat illness more likely, and increase orthostatic hypotension during exercise. Fever may accompany myocarditis or other infections that may make exercise dangerous. (*1, pp 143–147*)

25.7 (C) Smokers' risk is also higher for mouth, throat, esophageal, and cervical cancer. (*1, p 433*)

25.8 (B) Iron supplementation does not affect the guaiac test, although some iron supplements contain vitamin C in excess of 250 mg. (*1, p 248*)

25.9 (E) For mild hypertension, lifestyle modifications should be the initial treatment modality for the first 3 to 4 mo. (*1, pp 190–191*)

25.10 (E) Patients are advised to eat a normal diet and then fast for 12 h prior to cholesterol screening tests. Checking medications the patient is taking is important, as some (such as those listed) increase lipids. Screening should only be done on well patients whose weight is stable and who are not pregnant or nursing. The test is best done on a plasma sample. Patients should be in the sitting position for 5 min before the test sample is drawn to avoid orthostatic changes in lipid readings. (*1, pp 224–225*)

25.11 (D) Chlamydia is an organism that is difficult to culture. Any step in culturing that jeopardizes the accuracy of test results should be avoided or modified in order to minimize interference with result accuracy. (*1, p 288*)

25.12 (C) The patient is also at risk for HIV and hepatitis B. (*1, p 338*)

25.13 (D) The woman should be tested for hepatitis B surface antigen (HBsAg); if she tests positive, the man should begin the hepatitis B vaccine series and get a shot of HBIgG. If the woman is HBsAg negative, the man should begin the hepatitis B vaccine series only. (*1, p 342*)

25.14 (C) The eyes would not be in a conjugate gaze as with strabismus. (*2, p 218*)

25.15 (C) Normal levels of hemoglobin and hematocrit change for all the factors listed except ethnicity. (*1, p 5*)

25.16 (D) While DXA is the method currently favored for detection of osteoporosis, only quantitative computed tomography can distinguish between cortical and trabecular bone. (*1, pp 455–456*)

25.17 (A) Any of the immunization preparations may be used, although authorities recommend MMR given subcutaneously. The patient should be counseled not to become pregnant for 3 mo after immunization. The most common side effect is arthralgias, which occur in about 25% of adults immunized. (*1, pp 360–361*)

25.18 (E) Immunization against pneumococci is indicated in the elderly and in patients with surgical or functional asplenia. (*1, p 354*)

25.19 (D) According to the U.S. Task Force, screening for prostate cancer is controversial. The screening test of choice would be PSA (prostate-specific antigen), not acid phosphatase. Examination of the prostate by digital rectal exam is not a very sensitive test. There has not been shown to be a difference in the mortality of men of this patient's age group treated with radical therapy versus watchful waiting. (*1, pp 209–210*)

25.20 (C) Prior to 12 mo of age, a baby should receive breast milk or infant formula only. (*1, p 136*)

References

1. United States Office of Disease Prevention and Health Promotion: *Put Prevention into Practice: Clinician's Handbook of Preventive Services,* 2/e, McLean, VA, International Medical, 1998.

2. Bickley LS, Hoekelman RA: *Bates' Guide to Physical Examination and History Taking,* 7/e, Philadelphia, Lippincott, 1999.

26
Surgery

Salah Ayachi, PhD, PA-C, and Frank Ambriz, PA-C

DIRECTIONS (Questions 26.1–26.100): Each of the numbered items or incomplete statements in this chapter is followed by answers or completions of the statement. Select the **one** lettered answer or completion that is **best** in each case.

26.1 A patient's present and past medical history can have a significant effect on wound care. Which of the following would impact wound care the least?
  A. Diabetes
  B. Peripheral vascular disease
  C. Penicillin allergy
  D. Corticosteroid usage

26.2 Which is **NOT** a bedside indicator of shock?
  A. Warm extremities
  B. Tachycardia
  C. Peripheral vasoconstriction and cool extremities
  D. Oliguria

26.3 Which of the following historical data is **NOT** essential in evaluating a wound?
A. Nature of the traumatic episode
B. Current medications
C. Tetanus immunization
D. Prior travel to a foreign country

26.4 Prior to wound repair, you must
A. Perform a trauma-oriented neurologic exam
B. Cleanse the wound with alcohol
C. Administer oral antibiotics
D. Apply topical antibiotics

26.5 Factors that affect wound management include
A. Wound characteristics
B. Anatomical site
C. Underlying host conditions
D. All of the above

26.6 In which patient population is the risk of appendix perforation lowest?
A. Pregnant women
B. Patients under 10 years old
C. Patients over 50 years old
D. Adolescent boys

26.7 The fluid of choice for rapid volume replacement in the treatment of hemorrhagic shock is
A. Albumin
B. 5% dextrose in water
C. Normal saline
D. Lactated Ringer's

26.8 A patient with a hand wound that occurred 3 days earlier is seen in the ED with a laceration on the hypothenar eminence. Red streaking is seen on the ulnar side of the distal forearm. The patient reports being bitten by a cat. What is the most likely cause of the infection?
A. *Pasteurella multocida*
B. *Staphylococcus epidermidis*
C. *Pseudomonas aeruginosa*
D. *Trichomonas vaginalis*

26.9 The premalignant skin lesions that give rise to the least aggressive squamous cell carcinomas are
  A. Actinic keratoses
  B. Scars
  C. Chronic ulcers
  D. Chronic radiation dermatitis

26.10 Which of the following is **NOT** true of ventral hernias?
  A. The larger the fascial defect, the higher the recurrence rate.
  B. They are also known as direct inguinal hernias.
  C. They are usually due to poor surgical technique.
  D. Repair of large hernias calls for using nonabsorbable mesh.

26.11 For optimal wound healing with minimal scarring, you must
  A. Cleanse the dermal edges
  B. Debride the dermal edges
  C. Accurately approximate the dermal edges
  D. Do all the above

26.12 Which is **NOT** a toxic reaction to injection of local anesthetics?
  A. Wound contraction
  B. Cardiac vascular reaction
  C. Excitatory central nervous system effects
  D. Vasovagal syncope secondary to pain and anxiety

26.13 Which of the following is **NOT** true of decubitus ulcers (decubiti)?
  A. Treatment is usually prolonged and difficult.
  B. They result from prolonged pressure on the tissue.
  C. The first step in the management is to administer antibiotics.
  D. They are common in drug addicts.

26.14 To reduce the pain of injection, lidocaine is buffered with
  A. Epinephrine
  B. Sodium bicarbonate
  C. Demerol
  D. Heparin

26.15 Minimal pain during injection of local anesthetics is achieved by using needles of which gauge?
  A. 18
  B. 25
  C. 27
  D. 30

26.16 The wounds and lacerations that are least likely to develop infections are those involving
  A. The face and neck
  B. The perineum
  C. The hands and feet
  D. Jagged edges

26.17 A 49-year-old man, American Society of Anesthesiologists (ASA) class I, scheduled for an elective surgical procedure should have a(n)
  A. Electrocardiogram (ECG)
  B. ECG, chest x-ray (CXR), and hemoglobin and hematocrit (H&H)
  C. CXR, H&H, and urinalysis (UA)
  D. Complete blood count (CBC), CXR, and UA

26.18 Which is **NOT** a complication of the Trendelenburg position for surgical procedures?
  A. Atelectasis due to lung compression by abdominal viscera
  B. Overabduction of hip joints
  C. Masking of hypovolemia until the patient is returned to the supine position
  D. Cerebral edema due to increased central venous pressure

26.19 Which of the following statements about postoperative fever is **FALSE**?
  A. Fever due to atelectasis develops within the first 48 h after surgery.
  B. Fever due to infection develops after the second day following surgery.
  C. Fever due to intraabdominal abscess develops within the first 36 h after surgery.
  D. Fever due to catheter-related phlebitis develops after the second day following surgery.

26.20 Which of the following does **NOT** suggest a diagnosis of aortic coarctation?
   A. Increased pulse pressure in the lower extremities
   B. Diminished or absent femoral pulses
   C. Harsh systolic murmur heard in the back
   D. BP difference between upper and lower extremities or right and left arms

26.21 Which of the following radiographic findings is indicative of aortic coarctation?
   A. Ventricular hypertrophy
   B. Kerley B lines
   C. Mediastinal lucency
   D. Rib notching

26.22 Which signs and symptoms are **NOT** attributable to local anesthetic toxicity?
   A. Lightheadedness and facial paresthesias
   B. Shortened PR intervals
   C. Blurred vision and tinnitus
   D. Cardiac arrhythmias, especially in pregnant patients

26.23 Which hemostatic technique is most appropriate for repair of liver lacerations?
   A. Pressure (gauze pads)
   B. Topical agents
   C. Electrocautery
   D. Pledget-type sutures

26.24 Which of the following is **NOT** true about male breast cancer?
   A. It most commonly presents as a subareolar mass.
   B. It most commonly presents as invasive ductal carcinoma.
   C. It most commonly affects both breasts.
   D. It is treated in the same way as breast cancer in women.

26.25 Which is **NOT** true of right ventricular (RV) infarction?
   A. RV end-diastolic pressure decreases.
   B. Left ventricular end-diastolic size decreases.
   C. Treatment calls for nitrates.
   D. Dobutamine can be used for inotropic support.

26.26 Shock induces autonomic responses that serve to maintain perfusion pressure to vital organs. Which of the following is **NOT** a response to shock?
A. Constriction of venous capacitance vessels
B. Release of antidiuretic hormone
C. Decreased myocardial contractility
D. Release of vasoactive hormones including cortisol

26.27 In shock, pathologic events give rise to all the following clinical features **EXCEPT**
A. Hyperkalemia
B. Hyperglycemia
C. Metabolic acidosis
D. Hypernatremia

26.28 Presenting signs and symptoms of surgical wound infection include all of the following **EXCEPT**
A. Increasing pain at the incision site
B. Pallor
C. Drainage from the incision
D. Tenderness at the site

26.29 Factors influencing the development of infection include
A. Presence of foreign body
B. Decreased blood flow
C. Presence of necrotic tissue
D. All of the above

26.30 Which of the following does **NOT** increase the risk of infection?
A. Presence of dead space that prevents the delivery of phagocytic cells to bacterial foci
B. Poor approximation of tissue
C. Operations of long duration (10 h or longer)
D. Debridement of necrotic tissue

26.31 Lidocaine with epinephrine is contraindicated in the
A. Fingers
B. Toes
C. Penis
D. All the above

26.32 Which is true of physical findings in the elderly?
  A. Fewer than 25% of patients aged over 70 with perforated ulcer have abdominal rigidity.
  B. Appendicitis usually manifests in the left lower quadrant.
  C. Tachypnea is an indication the patient is out of shape.
  D. Abdominal distention is often due to intussusception.

26.33 The effect of epinephrine, when added to lidocaine, is to
  A. Produce vasoconstriction
  B. Decrease bleeding time
  C. Prolong effects of lidocaine
  D. Do all the above

26.34 Which is **NOT** a sign of peritoneal irritation?
  A. Rebound tenderness
  B. Voluntary guarding
  C. Homan sign
  D. Decreased or absent bowel sounds

26.35 Which is **NOT** a complication of laparoscopy?
  A. Pneumothorax
  B. Perforating injuries
  C. Infection
  D. Neurogenic shock

26.36 Which is **NOT** a typical sign of basilar skull fracture?
  A. Clear otorrhea or rhinorrhea
  B. Hemotympanum
  C. Battle sign
  D. Cullen sign

26.37 The most common symptom of pleural disease is
  A. Pleural effusion
  B. Pleuritic chest pain
  C. Empyema
  D. Hemothorax

26.38 The differential diagnosis of pleural effusion includes
   A. Tuberculosis
   B. Cancer
   C. Rheumatoid arthritis
   D. All of the above

Questions 26.39–26.42: Match the lettered items with the questions. Items may be used once, more than once, or not at all.
   A. Accumulation of air or gas in the pleura space
   B. Accumulation of blood in the pleura space
   C. Pleural effusion containing purulent material
   D. Endogenous fluid in the pleura space
   E. Air under the diaphragm

26.39 Pleural effusion

26.40 Empyema

26.41 Hemothorax

26.42 Pneumothorax

Questions 26.43–26.46: Match the lettered items with the questions. Items may be used once, more than once, or not at all.
   A. Occur most often in the second and third decades of life, with 60% of cases in men
   B. The most common primary malignant tumor of the chest wall
   C. Associated with systemic symptoms such as fever, malaise, and a painful, warm chest wall mass; x-ray findings show an "onion skin" calcification
   D. X-ray findings are "punched out" osteolytic lesions

26.43 Chondrosarcoma

26.44 Ewing's sarcoma

26.45 Myeloma

26.46 Osteosarcoma

26.47 Your surgical team is consulted for evaluation of a patient who is a cocaine smuggler and who swallowed small packets of cocaine in balloons. Your best approach is to
A. Perform immediate surgical removal
B. Give a laxative to expedite expulsion of the packets
C. Watch the patient carefully and see if the packets pass spontaneously
D. Give the patient psyllium (Metamucil) to cushion the packets

26.48 Ultrasonography is useful in evaluating abdominal pain suspected in all of the following **EXCEPT**
A. Ulcer disease
B. Abdominal masses
C. Appendicitis
D. Pregnancy

26.49 Disorders potentially amenable to splenectomy include all the following **EXCEPT**
A. Hereditary spherocytosis
B. Thalassemia major
C. Acquired hemolytic anemia
D. Infectious mononucleosis

26.50 Treatment of frostbite involves
A. Rewarming with water at 40 to 42°C until the area is thawed
B. Dressing and bandaging of affected parts
C. Systemic corticosteroids
D. Topical corticosteroids

26.51 Rupture of which of the following would **NOT** lead to pneumothorax?
A. Lung parenchyma
B. Esophagus
C. Chest wall
D. Thoracic aorta

26.52 Which of the following would **NOT** be found on the involved side in a case of pneumothorax?
  A. Chest pain
  B. Dyspnea
  C. Decreased breath sounds
  D. Increased vocal fremitus

26.53 The most frequent cause of intestinal obstruction is
  A. Strangulated groin hernia
  B. Adhesive band
  C. Malignancy
  D. Diverticulitis coli

26.54 A 44-year-old mother of two teenagers develops sudden abdominal pain. She has been treated for ulcers for the past 4 years. Physical exam reveals a rigid abdomen with severe pain radiating to the back and absent bowel sounds. The most likely diagnosis is
  A. Stone in the common bile duct
  B. Acute pancreatitis
  C. Perforated peptic ulcer
  D. Ectopic pregnancy

26.55 A 60-year-old diabetic man is found to have midepigastric abdominal pain and progressive jaundice with a palpable gallbladder. The most likely diagnosis is
  A. Pancreatic cancer
  B. Chronic cholecystitis
  C. Common bile duct stone
  D. Hepatitis

26.56 A 36-year-old male physician assistant student complains of severe rectal pain that awakens him in the middle of the night. The most likely diagnosis is
  A. Proctalgia fugax
  B. Amaurosis fugax
  C. Dysentery
  D. Ulcerative colitis

26.57 Post–head trauma syndrome may include
A. Headache
B. Insomnia
C. Personality changes
D. Restlessness
E. All of the above

26.58 The most important initial step in the management of severe trauma is to establish an airway. Following the establishment of an airway, you would proceed with
A. Evaluating the level of consciousness
B. Initiating diagnostic tests to evaluate possible intracranial hemorrhage
C. Obtaining lateral cervical spine films to rule out fracture
D. Establishing an IV line

26.59 A 55-year-old male smoker complains of left leg pain when walking. The pain is relieved with rest. Examination reveals a normal pulse in the femoral artery, but absent popliteal and pedal pulses. The surface skin of the left leg is normal. The possible diagnosis is
A. Phlebothrombosis
B. Femoral artery occlusion
C. Popliteal artery occlusion
D. Raynaud's disease

26.60 A patient with a head injury is brought to your office. You should now
A. Start an IV line
B. Establish an airway
C. Obtain a good history
D. Perform a good physical exam

26.61 The treatment of lymphangitis of the lower extremities is
A. Total excision
B. Antibiotics
C. Radiation
D. Cryosurgery

26.62 Sutures used to approximate the edges of the cartilage in the pinna of the ear should be removed in
  A. 3 to 5 days
  B. 7 to 10 days
  C. 10 to 14 days
  D. None of the above

26.63 A 38-year-old woman develops a temperature of 38.2°C 24 h following cholecystectomy. She has no complaints and her physical exam is unremarkable. The most appropriate management of this patient would be to
  A. Start her on antibiotics
  B. Do urine, sputum, and blood cultures
  C. Continue observation
  D. Take her back for exploratory surgery

26.64 The most consistent finding in acute cholecystitis is
  A. Pain and tenderness in the upper right quadrant
  B. Elevated serum enzymes
  C. Elevated white blood count
  D. Fever

26.65 Which of the following statements about testicular torsion is **NOT** true?
  A. It can present with nausea, vomiting, and fever.
  B. It is a twisting of the testis in its cord.
  C. Immediate surgical intervention is advised when torsion is suspected.
  D. It usually presents with penile discharge.

26.66 The most common cause of abdominal pain in patients over 65 years of age who present to the emergency department is
  A. Acute gastroenteritis
  B. Acute cholecystitis
  C. Abdominal anergies
  D. Acute myocardial infarction

26.67 Suture size is defined by the number of zeroes. Which of the following is the smallest suture?
A. 6-0 (000000)
B. 5-0 (00000)
C. 3-0 (000)
D. 2-0 (00)

26.68 The process of wound healing is divided into four stages, which include all the following **EXCEPT**
A. Inflammation
B. Fibroblast proliferation
C. Contraction
D. Regeneration
E. Remolding

26.69 Wound healing by primary intention involves wounds that are
A. Not closed with sutures
B. Closed by contraction and epithelialization
C. Closed with sutures
D. Infected and patched open
E. Left open for a period of time and sutured at a later date

26.70 Wound healing by secondary intention involves all wounds **EXCEPT** those
A. Not closed with sutures
B. Closed by contraction and epithelialization
C. Closed with sutures
D. Infected and patched open
E. Left open for a period of time and then sutured at a later date

26.71 In wound healing by tertiary intent, the wound is
A. Not closed with sutures
B. Closed by contraction and epithelialization
C. Closed with sutures
D. Infected and patched open
E. Left open for a period of time and then sutured at a later date

26.72 The choice of appropriate suture material is based on the
   A. Location and extent of the laceration
   B. Strength of the tissue
   C. Preference of the clinician
   D. A and B
   E. A, B, and C

26.73 The suture material most appropriate for the face is
   A. 3-0 silk
   B. 4-0 nylon
   C. 5-0 or 6-0 nylon or prolene
   D. 2-0 silk

26.74 The suture most appropriate for the scalp is
   A. 3-0 nylon
   B. 3-0 absorbable suture
   C. 4-0 silk
   D. 6-0 nylon

26.75 Suture marks ("tracks") are the result of
   A. Excessive tension on the tissue
   B. Leaving the suture in too long
   C. Excess povidone-iodine (Betadine) to clean the wound
   D. A and B only

26.76 Concerning preoperative evaluation, which of the following is **NOT** true?
   A. A thorough and detailed history and physical exam are the most important factors in evaluating the surgical patient.
   B. Electrocardiogram is necessary to rule out ischemic heart disease prior to surgery.
   C. H/H should be done on all patients undergoing surgery.
   D. Urinalysis is unlikely to contribute to the care of the patient.

26.77 In surgical patients, the majority of pulmonary emboli go unrecognized because other conditions present in a similar way. Which does **NOT**?
   A. Congestive heart failure
   B. Pneumonia

C. Atelectasis
D. Hypertension

26.78 The most common infections acquired in the hospital involve
A. The urinary tract
B. The respiratory tract
C. Wounds
D. All of the above

26.79 Common early signs of gas-forming soft tissue infection include
A. Pain
B. Mental disorientation
C. Tachycardia
D. All of the above

26.80 Which is **NOT** a principle of preoperative antibiotic prophylaxis?
A. Select the antibiotic(s) most appropriate for the expected pathogens.
B. Use antibiotics only if the benefit outweighs the risk of their use.
C. Give the appropriate dose of antibiotic(s) at the appropriate time(s).
D. Give only first-line antibiotics for the expected pathogens.

26.81 Factors implicated in the etiology of pressure sores include
A. Pressure
B. Ischemia
C. Denervation
D. A and B
E. A, B, and C

26.82 Which is an absolute indication for exploratory laparotomy, even in a patient who is asymptomatic?
A. Free air under the diaphragm on plain x-ray
B. Presence of calculi in the gallbladder on plain x-ray
C. Leucocytosis of 17,500 or greater with left shift
D. Air in the large bowel on plain x-ray

26.83 Neurologic focal deficits associated with TIAs (numbness, paresthesias, weakness)
   A. Last less than 24 h and often resolve within 1 h
   B. Last longer than 24 h, but less than 48 h
   C. Are chronic, often lasting for years
   D. Are associated with anterior cruciate ligament tears

26.84 A patient who presents with rapid onset of severe, constant abdominal pain and amenorrhea or abnormal uterine bleeding
   A. Should be considered to have an ectopic pregnancy until proven otherwise
   B. Is in no immediate danger
   C. Should have immediate culdocentesis
   D. Should be treated for acute salpingitis

26.85 Diagnostic studies that must be done immediately when assessing a patient with acute abdomen include all of the following **EXCEPT**
   A. Chest radiography
   B. Arterial blood gases (ABGs)
   C. Liver function enzymes
   D. Hematocrit

26.86 Elderly patients with diabetes are prone to developing serious postoperative complications. Which of the following is related to autonomic neuropathy?
   A. Hypoglycemia
   B. Hypotension
   C. Myocardial infarction
   D. Volume overload

26.87 In diabetics, wound flora are typically mixed. Which organism(s) would you suspect in patients with severe infections that do not respond to treatment with antibacterials?
   A. *Staphylococcus aureus*
   B. *Escherichia coli*
   C. *P. aeruginosa*
   D. *Candida albicans*

26.88 Which of the following conditions causes femoral head avascular necrosis via bone marrow sludging?
A. Sickle cell disease
B. Corticosteroid use
C. Alcohol abuse
D. Hyperlipidemia

26.89 Which is true of avascular necrosis (AVN) of the femoral head?
A. The contralateral hip is involved in 20% to 25% of cases.
B. It is a disease of the elderly.
C. The most definitive diagnostic procedure is biopsy.
D. Arthrodesis is a viable surgical option in these cases.

26.90 Which is not true of abdominal aortic aneurysms (AAAs)?
A. African American males have a higher incidence of AAAs than do white males.
B. The rate is nearly 12 times higher in first-degree relatives of patients with AAAs.
C. Poor oxygenation and nutrition of the distal aorta play an important role.
D. Back pain or abdominal pain is the most commonly reported complaint in symptomatic patients.

26.91 The "gold standard" (Ross method) in replacement of aortic valve (AV) with bioprosthesis uses
A. Cadaver AV
B. Porcine AV
C. Mechanical AV
D. Autograft of pulmonic valve

26.92 Which is **NOT** an alternative to total knee replacement surgery in a patient with osteoarthritis?
A. Hyaluronic acid injections
B. Chondrocyte transplantation
C. Osteochondral fixation
D. Synovectomy

26.93 Which of the following is the hollow viscus most commonly injured during laparoscopic cholecystectomy?
A. Small intestine
B. Colon
C. Stomach
D. Abdominal aorta

26.94 Which of the following symptoms of appendicitis is reported most frequently?
A. Anorexia
B. Abdominal pain
C. Nausea/vomiting
D. Fever/chills

26.95 The most common cause of acute renal failure in both medical and surgical patients is
A. Hypovolemia
B. Aminoglycoside toxicity
C. Urethral swelling after injury
D. Disruption of urinary drainage

26.96 Which of the following diagnostic methods of evaluating patients with possible abdominal injury is accurate, noninvasive, and practical?
A. Computed tomography
B. Ultrasound
C. Peritoneal lavage
D. MRI

26.97 Which method of nonsurgical treatment of hemorrhoids has fewer and less severe complications?
A. Rubber band ligation
B. Injection sclerotherapy
C. Infrared coagulation
D. Cryotherapy

26.98 Your patient has a lesion of his left 4th toe that you suspect to be melanoma. Your exam reveals painful inguinal nodes. Which of the following is the best method of managing this patient?

A. Chemotherapy
B. Surgical resection
C. Radiotherapy
D. All of the above

26.99 Which of the following is the number one indication for hysterectomy?
A. Uterine leiomyomas
B. Dysfunctional uterine bleeding
C. Genital prolapse
D. Chronic pelvic pain

26.100 In which of the following hernias is a loop of intestine most likely to become incarcerated?
A. Umbilical hernia
B. Ventral hernia
C. Femoral hernia
D. Indirect inguinal hernia

Surgery

Answers and Discussion

26.1 (C) Conditions such as diabetes and peripheral vascular disease can increase the risk of wound infection and cause delayed or poor healing. It is well known that corticosteroids adversely affect the normal healing process. Allergies to antibiotics should not delay wound healing or increase the risk of infection. (*1, p 282*)

26.2 (A) Warm extremities without hypotension are an indicator of good circulation. Tachycardia, peripheral vasoconstriction and cool extremities, and oliguria are markers of hypoperfusion. (*2, pp 107–108*)

26.3 (D) Wounds and lacerations are often the result of or the cause of systemic problems and illness. Patients who fall and sustain minor injuries may need to be questioned and examined for causes of syncope. (*1, p 282*)

26.4 (A) In addition to wound repair, a trauma-oriented neurological exam is often necessary. (*1, p 282*)

26.5 (D) The combination of wound characteristics, anatomic site, and underlying host conditions affects the management of every wound. Each patient is unique and requires individualized treatment. (*1, p 282*)

26.6 (D) The patient population with the lowest risk of appendix perforation is adolescents. The risk in patients under 10 or over 50 can be as high as 75% or higher. In the case of pregnant patients, the risk of perforation is due to delayed diagnosis. (*3, pp 611–612; 2, pp 242–244*)

26.7 (D) In patients with hypovolemic shock, lactated Ringer's should be used for initial resuscitation even when blood is available. Blood should be withheld until bleeding has been controlled. (*3, p 188*)

26.8 (A) Cat bites cause infection via *P. multocida,* which responds to penicillin. (*1, p 335*)

26.9 (A) Squamous cell carcinomas that develop from actinic keratoses are the least aggressive. (*3, pp 1149–1150*)

26.10 (B) Ventral hernias, also referred to as incisional hernias, can be due to many factors including poor technique, postoperative wound infection, and pulmonary complications resulting in coughing. Generally, the larger the hernia, the higher the likelihood of recurrence and the need for using nonabsorbable mesh for repair. (*3, pp 720–721*)

26.11 (D) Every effort is made to cleanse, judiciously debride, and accurately approximate the dermal edges to allow for optimal wound healing with minimal scar formation. (*1, p 285*)

26.12 (A) The most common reaction to local anesthetic is vasovagal syncope. Cardiovascular reactions include hypotension and bradycardia. The excitatory phenomenon in the central nervous system can culminate in seizure activity. (*3, pp 174–185*)

26.13 (C) The first important step in treating decubiti is to incise and drain infected spaces or necrotic areas. (*3, p 90*)

26.14 (B) A promising new approach to reducing the pain of local anesthetic infiltrate is to add sodium bicarbonate buffer to lidocaine. The rationale is that the relatively acidic pH of lidocaine is the cause of the pain. (*1, p 259*)

26.15 (D) When injecting local anesthetics, the smallest gauge (30 g) is recommended for minimum pain. (*1, p 259*)

26.16 (A) The face and neck have a very high blood supply and are less likely to develop infections. Wounds that are more complex or that involve the perineum, hands, or feet are more prone to be infected. (*1, p 283*)

26.17 (A) Preoperative laboratory tests required for elective surgery on a 49-year-old man without systemic disease (ASA-I) are limited to ECG. In the case of older men (over 60) who are ASA-I, H&H, CXR, BUN, glucose, and ECG are required. (*4, p 4*)

26.18 (B) Overabduction of the hip joints is a complication of the lithotomy position. (*4, p 9*)

26.19 (C) Patients who have normal convalescence rarely have fever after the first week. Fever due to intraabdominal abscesses generally develops after the first postoperative week. (*3, p 38*)

26.20 (A) Pulse pressure is decreased in the lower extremities. (*3, pp 388–389*)

26.21 (D) Rib notching is due to erosions on the underside of the ribs caused by enlargement and tortuosity of intercostal vessels produced as a result of collateral circulation. (*5, pp 428–429*)

26.22 (B) PR intervals are prolonged in local anesthetic toxicity, and so are conduction times and QRS intervals. With higher doses, heart blocks develop. (*1, p 258*)

26.23 (D) Pledget-type sutures, also used with spleen lacerations, are used in cases of liver lacerations in order to reduce the chances of sutures cutting through the tissues. (*4, pp 74–84*)

26.24 (C) Male breast cancer most commonly affects only one breast. (*6, pp 284–293*)

26.25 (C) With RV infarction, both RV end-diastolic pressure and LV end-diastolic size decrease, and inotropic support (with dobutamine) becomes necessary. However, nitrates (and other drugs that reduce preload) are not recommended because they produce hemodynamic derangements. (*1, p 372*)

26.26 (C) The autonomic responses to shock are mediated by catecholamines that directly or indirectly cause venoconstriction, activate the renin-angiotensin-aldosterone system and release of antidiuretic hormone, and increase myocardial contractility. Cortisol is released in response to the stress of shock. (*1, p 215*)

26.27 (D) The metabolic derangements associated with shock include hyponatremia, which results from leakage of sodium into the cells that are unable to maintain their selective permeability. (*1, p 216*)

26.28 (D) Pain, tenderness, and edema are indicative of wound infection. Erythema, not pallor, is the other feature. (*1, p 595*)

26.29 (D) Foreign bodies (e.g., sutures, drains, or grafts), decreased blood flow, and necrotic tissue all contribute to the development of infection. (*1, p 323*)

26.30 (D) The presence of necrotic tissue adds to the risk for infection. Debriding the necrotic tissue reduces the risk. (*2, pp 146–160*)

26.31 (D) Because epinephrine is a vasoconstrictor, the possibility of ischemic necrosis makes its use with lidocaine in the areas mentioned a contraindication. (*1, p 257*)

26.32 (A) Disease presentation in the elderly may differ from that in younger adults, thus confounding the clinical picture and resulting in missed diagnoses. In the elderly, abdominal distention more than likely means obstruction, tachypnea indicates respiratory and/or cardiovascular insufficiency, and appendicitis localizes to the RLQ. (*1, pp 516–517*)

26.33 (D)   Epinephrine is meant to constrict the small vessels and thus decrease bleeding and decrease the washout of the lidocaine from the area, prolonging the effect of lidocaine. (*1, p 257*)

26.34 (C)   All the signs listed indicate peritoneal irritation except the Homan sign, which is more indicative of calf tenderness with suspected deep vein thrombosis. (*3, pp 318–324*)

26.35 (D)   Pneumothorax, bleeding, perforated injuries, infection, intestinal injuries, solid organ injury, and vascular injury are all complications that can arise from laparoscopy. (*1, p 598*)

26.36 (D)   Clear rhinorrhea, hemotympanum, the Battle sign, and "raccoon eyes" could all be signs of skull fracture. (*4, p 245; 3, p 869*)

26.37 (B)   The most common complaint in pleural disease is pleuritic pain, a chest pain associated with respiratory exertion that sometimes reflexively inhibits respiration. (*4, p 102*)

26.38 (D)   Included in the differential diagnosis of pleural effusion are tuberculosis, cancer, and rheumatoid arthritis, along with congestive heart failure, pneumonia, and pulmonary embolism. (*3, p 603*)

26.39–26.42 (D), (C), (B), (A)   Pleural effusion denotes fluid in the pleural space. A more exact term is used when the character of the fluid is known. Air, not fluid, is in the pleural space in pneumothorax. (*3, pp 603–604*)

26.43 (B)   About 15% to 20% of all skeletal chondrosarcomas occur in the ribs and sternum. Skeletal chondrosarcoma is the most common malignant tumor of the chest wall. (*5, pp 252–253*)

26.44 (C)   Ewing's sarcoma is associated with systemic symptoms such as fever, malaise, and chest pain. These tumors are highly malignant, and evidence of skeletal lesion on x-ray ("onion skin") is present in 30% to 75% of patients when first seen. (*5, pp 252–253*)

26.45 (D) Tumors are found as a manifestation of systemic multiple myeloma. (*5, pp 252–253*)

26.46 (A) Osteosarcoma is more malignant than chondrosarcoma, and the prognosis is poor. X-ray findings of bone destruction and recalcification at right angles to the bony cortex give the "sunburst" appearance. (*5, pp 252–253*)

26.47 (C) Rupture of one packet of cocaine, particularly high-grade material, can be fatal. Attempts at endoscopic removal run the risk of rupture of the bags and should be considered unsafe. If it appears the packets may be passed spontaneously, the patient may be observed. Otherwise, surgical removal is indicated. (*5, pp 293–294; 1, p 1114*)

26.48 (A) Ultrasonography has a diagnostic sensitivity of about 80% for acute appendicitis. It is useful in investigating abdominal masses and in evaluating patients presenting with features of pelvic inflammatory disease or possible pregnancy. (*4, p 117*)

26.49 (D) All the conditions listed may necessitate removal of the spleen. The exception is infectious mononucleosis, where splenomegaly resolves spontaneously if there are no complications such as rupture due to injury from blunt trauma. (*4, p 599*)

26.50 (A) Frostbite is treated by rewarming with water at 40 to 42°C until the area is thawed. The affected parts are elevated; trauma should be prevented. Corticosteroids should be avoided. (*4, pp 708–709*)

26.51 (D) Pneumothorax may be caused by rupture of the esophagus, the lung parenchyma, or the chest wall itself. Rupture of the thoracic aorta, for whatever reason, without involvement of other systems usually results in fatal hemothorax. (*3, pp 333–334, 377–380*)

26.52 (D)   Chest pain, dyspnea, and decreased breath sounds on the involved side all can be noted with pneumothorax, but fremitus (tactile and vocal) is decreased. (*3, pp 333–334*)

26.53 (B)   Strangulated groin hernia is the second most frequent cause of intestinal obstruction; neoplasm of the bowel is third. Diverticulitis coli is also seen, but usually in the older age group. Adhesive bandages are the most common cause for all age groups. (*3, p 624*)

26.54 (C)   Sudden onset of severe abdominal pain and past history of ulcer point to likely perforation. A stone in the common bile duct would lead to jaundice and present with a history of gradual onset of crampy abdominal pain. (*3, pp 492–494*)

26.55 (A)   Carcinoma of the pancreatic head is frequently found in diabetic men over 60 years of age. (*3, pp 586–589*)

26.56 (A)   Proctalgia fugax is a severe, spasmodic rectal pain lasting a few minutes, whose cause is unknown. It is reported in patients who are overworked and anxious. (*3, p 708*)

26.57 (E)   All the complaints listed may present after a head injury. (*3, p 821*)

26.58 (A)   In the management of severe trauma, following the establishment of an airway, the level of consciousness, conditions of the pupils, and vital signs should be evaluated, and bleeding sites should be identified and controlled. (*3, p 821*)

26.59 (C)   Occlusion of the popliteal artery leads to severe claudication. Femoral artery occlusion would result in absent common femoral pulses. (*3, p 750*)

26.60 (B)   The most important initial step in the management of any severe trauma is the establishment of an airway. (*3, p 821*)

26.61 (B)   Lymphangitis is frequently caused by streptococci, and should be treated with appropriate antibiotics. (*3, pp 94–101*)

26.62 (D) Sutures used to repair cartilage in the ear pinna should not be removed. Sutures placed in the skin may be removed in about 5 days. (*1, p 304*)

26.63 (C) Postoperative fever within the first 24 h of surgery without a source can be attributed to the stress response to the surgical procedure. Be careful to rule out the number one cause of fever—atelectasis. (*1, pp 592–593*)

26.64 (A) Elevated white cell counts may be found in acute cholecystitis, but the most consistent finding is right upper quadrant pain and tenderness. (*1, p 577*)

26.65 (D) Torsion of the spermatic cord is a surgical emergency. Clinical findings can include pain, nausea, vomiting, and fever. The cremasteric reflex is absent on the affected side. (*1, p 635*)

26.66 (B) Acute cholecystitis is by far the most common cause of abdominal pain in patients over 65 years old who present to the ED. (*1, p 517*)

26.67 (A) The higher the number (i.e., the more zeroes), the smaller the suture. (*1, pp 287–288*)

26.68 (D) Wound healing occurs generally in four stages: inflammation, fibroblast proliferation, contraction, and then remolding. (*3, pp 80–93*)

26.69–26.71 (C), (C), (E) Wound healing can be primary (routine primary suturing) or secondary (wound not closed by sutures, but rather closed by contraction and epithelialization). Tertiary intent, in which the wound is left intentionally open and closed at a later date, is also called delayed primary closure. (*3, pp 80–93*)

26.72 (E) The choice of the appropriate suture material is based on many factors, including location and extent of the laceration, strength of the tissue, and preference of the clinician. (*1, pp 287–288*)

26.73–26.74 (C), (A)   As a general guideline, face lacerations should be closed with 5-0 or 6-0 nylon or prolene when cosmetic concerns are important. Scalp lacerations should be closed with 3-0 nylon, and trunk or extremities should require 4-0 or 5-0 nylon. (*1, p 298*)

26.75 (D)   Suture marks are a result of excessive tension on the tissue or of leaving sutures in too long. (*5, pp 74–85*)

26.76 (B)   ECG is a poor predictor of ischemic heart disease. (*5, pp 82–84*)

26.77 (D)   CHF and pneumonia are particularly common in the postoperative period. Atelectasis is also common. Patients with PE all present with dyspnea. The presence of a sudden, unexplained drop in blood pressure strongly suggests pulmonary embolism. (*5, pp 450–454; 3, pp 26–27*)

26.78 (A)   All of the infections mentioned are commonly acquired in the hospital. Most urinary tract infections may be due to instrumentation (catheters). Pneumonia is the leading cause of infection-related death. Hospital-acquired pneumonias are often due to aerobic gram-negative bacteria. (*5, pp 17–27*)

26.79 (B)   Gas production causes crepitus and is often accompanied by hypotension, mental confusion, and multiple organ system failure. (*5, pp 17–27*)

26.80 (D)   First-line antibiotics should not be given as prophylactic agents. There is always the concern and risk of resistance development as well as the use of inappropriate drugs and doses. (*4, p 103; 1, pp 125–126*)

26.81 (E)   When pressure on the skin overlying a bone exceeds capillary pressure, ischemic necrosis develops. There is also evidence that local factors in denervated skin predispose to pressure breakdown. (*3, p 1160*)

26.82 (A)   A radiologic finding of free gas under the hemidiaphragm is an indication for urgent operation even before a diagnosis is established. (*3, p 451*)

26.83 (A) By convention, the arbitrary limit of a TIA is 24 h. Most TIAs last only minutes. (*3, p 762*)

26.84 (A) Rapid-onset severe and constant pain may be due to acute pancreatitis, mesenteric thrombosis, or ectopic pregnancy. A history of amenorrhea in a female of reproductive age should alert you to the likelihood of ectopic pregnancy causing the acute surgical abdomen. (*3, pp 441–452*)

26.85 (C) Liver enzyme levels may be performed on the same day to ascertain whether the acute abdomen is surgical or medical and to ascertain the extent of parenchymal disease. Chest x-ray, hematocrit, ABGs, and other tests including abdominal radiography, occult blood, cross-matching, and others must be performed immediately. (*3, pp 441–452*)

26.86 (B) Hypotension is ascribable to autonomic nervous system dysfunction associated with diabetes. Hypoglycemia develops in fasted patients given insulin and in those treated with beta blockers. Myocardial infarction is a complication in both diabetics and nondiabetics. Hypervolemia is related to diabetic nephropathy. (*7, p 10*)

26.87 (D) Antibiotic coverage in diabetics should include anaerobic bacteria, gram-negative enteric bacteria, and *S. aureus* to prevent diabetic ulceration in the lower extremities. If treatment is not successful, the clinician should suspect other infectious agents (e.g., candida). (*7, p 14*)

26.88 (A) Sickled cells cause sludging in the bone marrow and vessels, thus compromising the blood supply to the femoral head and resulting in its necrosis. (*8, pp 13–25*)

26.89 (C) Bone biopsy is the most accurate method of diagnosing AVN, but it is invasive. Most AVN victims are relatively young (one study cited in this reference notes the average age as 45 years). Arthrodesis (joint fixation) is contraindicated because AVN is bilateral in 50% to 80% of cases. (*8, pp 14–19*)

26.90 (A) White males have twice the incidence of AAAs as do African American males. First-degree relatives of patients with AAAs have a 12-fold higher risk of developing the condition, which is thought to be at least partly due to failure of the vasa vasorum resulting in decreased oxygenation of the distal aorta and formation of aneurysms. (*9, pp 20–24*)

26.91 (D) The Ross method, initiated by Donald Ross in 1962, calls for using the patient's own pulmonic valve to replace the diseased aortic valve. (*10, pp 919–924*)

26.92 (D) Of the methods listed, synovectomy is not an alternative to TKA. Viable options call for transplanting chondrocytes, osteochondral fixation, or injection of hyaluronic acid (a proteoglycan similar to bone matrix) into the arthritic joint. (*11, pp 1–11*)

26.93 (A) The small intestine is the most commonly injured viscus. Damage may be due to needle punctures, thermal injury from electrocautery, or retraction tears. Such injuries generally are not recognized until patients develop sepsis, fistulas, abscesses, or peritonitis. (*12, pp 813–823*)

26.94 (B) Abdominal pain is reported by 98% of patients with appendicitis, anorexia by 70%, nausea and vomiting by 67%, and fever and chills by only 20%. (*13, pp 2005–2011*)

26.95 (A) Hypovolemia is the most common cause of acute renal failure (ARF). (*14, pp 12–17*)

26.96 (B) Ultrasound has been shown to be an accurate method of evaluating patients in the emergency department for possible abdominal injury. It can be easily repeated at the bedside, is available in many more areas, and requires less training than the other methods listed. It has been used successfully in Europe for many years. (*15, pp 323–330*)

26.97 (C) In a retrospective study of 863 patients, infrared photocoagulation was associated with both fewer and less severe complications including pain, bleeding, and recurrence. (*16, pp 1601–1606*)

26.98 (B) Surgical resection is considered superior to any other available therapy for metastatic melanoma. (*17, pp 413–417*)

26.99 (A) Leiomyomas (fibroids) are the reason for hysterectomy in some 30% of cases. Chronic pelvic pain is the preoperative indication for hysterectomy in only 10% of cases. (*18, pp 856–860*)

26.100 (D) Femoral hernias are likely to incarcerate, but are uncommon. Ventral and umbilical hernias usually have wide openings. The most likely to incarcerate is the indirect inguinal hernia. (*1, pp 543–547*)

References

1. Tintinalli JE, Kelen GD, Stapzcynski: *Emergency Medicine: A Comprehensive Study Guide,* 5/e, New York, McGraw-Hill, 2000.

2. Lawrence PF, Bell RM, Dayton MT (eds): *Essentials of General Surgery,* 3/e, Philadelphia, Lippincott, 2000.

3. Way LW (ed): *Current Surgical Diagnosis & Treatment,* 10/e, Norwalk, CT, Appleton & Lange, 1994.

4. Deitch EA (ed): *Tools of the Trade and Rules of the Road— A Surgical Guide,* Philadelphia, Lippincott-Raven, 1997.

5. Davis JH, Foster RS, Gamelli RL: *Essentials of Clinical Surgery,* St. Louis, Mosby-Year Book, 1991.

6. Pollock RE (ed): *Breast Cancer,* MD Anderson Solid Tumor Oncology Series, New York, Springer, 1999.

7. Korber KE, Derman GH: Managing older diabetic patients undergoing surgery. *Surg Physician Assist* 5(4):10–14, 1999.

8. Shinnick JP: Diagnosing and management of nontraumatic avascular necrosis of the femoral head. *Surg Physician Assist* 6(2):14–19, 2000.

9. Ghandi RH, Snyder SO: Abdominal aortic aneurysm: Diagnosis and management. *Surg Physician Assist* 1(3):20–24, 1995.

10. Gross C, Harringer W, Beran H, et al: Aortic valve replacement: Is the stentless xenograft an alternative to the homograft? Midterm results. *Ann Thorac Surg* 68:919–924, 1999.

11. Vangsness CT; Complex topics in knee surgery: Overview of treatment options for arthritis in the active patient. *Clin Sports Med* 18(1):1–11, 1999.

12. Callery MP, Strasberg SM, Soper NJ: Complications of laparoscopic general surgery. *Gastrointest Endoscopy Clin North Am* 6(2):423–448, 1996.

13. Greenfield RH, Henneman PL: *Emergency Medicine Concepts and Clinical Practice,* 4/e, St. Louis, Mosby, 1998.

14. Pinevich AJ, Calhoun BC: Acute renal failure in trauma patients. *Surg Physician Assist* 5(9):12–17, 1999.

15. Porter RS, Nester BA, Dalsey WC, et al: Use of ultrasound to determine need for laparotomy in trauma patients. *Ann Emerg Med* 29:323–330, 1997.

16. Johanson JF, Rimm A: Optimal nonsurgical treatment of hemorrhoids: A comparative analysis of infrared coagulation, rubber ligation, and injection sclerotherapy. *J Gastroenterol* 87(11):1601–1606, 1992.

17. Fletcher WS, Pommier RF, Lum S, Wilmarth TJ: Surgical treatment of metastatic melanoma. *Am J Surg* 175:413–417, 1998.

18. Carlson KJ, Nichols DH, Schiff I: Current concepts: Indications for hysterectomy. *New Engl J Med* 328(12):856–860, 1993.